THE WHYS AND WHEREFORES OF CORPORATE PRACTICE

THE WHYS AND WHEREFORES OF CORPORATE PRACTICE

SHELDON H. GORLICK, J.D.
EDITOR AND PRINCIPAL AUTHOR

THIRD EDITION

MEDICAL ECONOMICS COMPANY
Book Division
Oradell, New Jersey

Design by Al Foti

ISBN 0-87489-209-0

Medical Economics Company
Oradell, New Jersey 07649

Printed in the United States of America

First Edition April, 1971
Second Edition July, 1976
Third Edition June, 1978

CONTENTS

publisher's NOTE

The content of this book is based on material first published in various issues of Medical Economics magazine. It also includes all relevant material from an earlier booklet "Now You Can Incorporate" and the previous versions of this book. While addressed to physicians, it applies in general to most professional and small-business men.

About the author:
Dividing his time between the editorial staff of Medical Economics magazine and his private legal practice, Sheldon H. Gorlick has been actively involved with pension and profit-sharing programs and professional corporations for over 15 years. A member of the New York and New Jersey bars, he has formed numerous professional corporations in those states. He also has spoken before thousands of physicians and counseled individuals and groups of doctors throughout the country. He has been a member of the Medical Economics staff since 1961.

1 Is incorporation worth it? 19 out of 20 say yes

Incorporation: It's attracted Internal Revenue Service agents like bees to the blossoms; a lot of tax-sheltered corporate retirement money has gone down the drain in the stock market; and there have even been divorces caused by a drop in take-home pay. But be not dismayed—those factors pale into insignificance when compared to the advantages, according to a Medical Economics survey of incorporated doctors.

When the survey's 628 responses were tabulated, they showed an overwhelming 95 per cent of physicians are happy they decided to incorporate their practices. Those 628 represent a response rate of better than 50 per cent; in all, 1,148 questionnaires were sent out to office-based doctors who indicated in previous Medical Economics surveys that they were incorporated.

The survey covers corporations of various sizes in all

geographical areas of the country, and it reveals lessons of importance for both the doctor who's already incorporated and the one who may be considering a switch from self-employment. (For some idea of the doctors who've already incorporated, see the box on pages 18-19.) For example, if you're one considering incorporation, make sure that you've budgeted for a drop in take-home pay. Remember, while you do save taxes through the deductions you get for the money you put away in a retirement plan, you still have to put the money away.

Here's another tip. Before and after incorporation, a key element of success is the advice you get. Choose your lawyer and accountant carefully, and if you're not satisfied later, change.

Most important, don't try for a killing with your pension and profit-sharing investments. The experience of incorporated doctors over the long pull shows the slow and sure way is best.

Now let's turn to the most important results of the survey, together with the analysis and advice of physicians now working in corporate practices. You're sure to benefit from their experiences.

Are your pension and/or profit-sharing plans growing as you expected? Yes, 46% No, 54%

While the vagaries of the stock market are responsible for most of the disappointment, many respondents blame their advisers for not shifting in time. A Tennessee doctor, for instance, reports that his eight-man group's fund lost $52,000 in one year. A Milwaukee physician says that the retirement fund for his five-man corporation has suffered a 40 per cent loss. Who's to blame for such heavy losses?

Many respondents indicate that the professional help they've gotten with their investments has failed to protect their nest eggs.

For instance, a Toledo physician is furious about the advice he's gotten, saying, "That damn fool at the bank doesn't know any more than I do about investing!"

Judging from survey responses, only a small percentage of doctors have taken advantage of the high interest rates available on bonds and short-term bills and notes in recent years.

But some of the respondents credit their agility in moving in response to the changing investment climate with heading off losses. They moved out of stocks before the prices dropped, and into short-term Treasury bills and corporate notes, thus managing to hold on to their gains. While many investment-wise doctors have sidestepped any problems by having 100 per cent of their retirement funds in bonds, it remains to be seen whether such an unbalanced investment policy will continue to be successful.

After incorporating, have you experienced any problems because of reduced take-home pay? Yes, 28% No, 72%

For the most part, answers indicating problems here reflect initial incorporating experience. And most of those say they've since ironed out their problems. In the words of a Garden City, N.Y., G.P.: "Although I had to make an adjustment in my budget, I like drawing a salary very much now." One way to avoid a financial crunch, many indicate, is to have a cash cushion to help ride out periods when corporate expenses are especially heavy.

A number of respondents say that they haven't experienced any drop at all in current income. Some, like one Peoria, Ill., M.D., state simply that "volume continues to increase" with retirement-plan savings coming out of the gains in earnings.

Other respondents don't mind an income reduction because the corporation now picks up and tax-deducts many expenses that formerly had to be paid out of after-tax money. A 43-year-old Rochester, N.Y., doctor balanced his reduction by shifting $8,000 in life and disability insurance premiums to the corporation.

Expanding volume and shifting insurance premiums are ways to take the teeth out of an income reduction, but many doctors simply aren't in a position to take advantage of them. In that case, the only thing to do is assume a philosophical attitude similar to that of the Flemington, N.J., physician who writes: "You know you'll take home less, so you plan for it." Still in some cases, the financial problems never really get worked out, and years after incorporating those doctors are grumbling about their financial difficulties. Perhaps they would have complained even if they hadn't incorporated.

In some cases, though, loss of income can cause serious problems. For example, a doctor in a small town in Pennsylvania reports that because of the wife's unwillingness or inability to comprehend why she had less money to spend after her husband incorporated, the couple ended up getting divorced. Several other physicians reported similar difficulties leading to divorce.

Do you find it an advantage to be on salary with income and Social Security taxes withheld? Yes, 83% No, 17%

Most respondents explain that they like being on the pay-as-you-go system because it's "more orderly" or that it "helps me live within my means." But an M.D. from Elmira, N.Y., comes through loud and clear: "This was the first time in 14 years that April wasn't a catastrophe," he says in explaining the advantages of having his tax bill current. Echoing that idea, a Eugene, Ore., doctor comments, "Now April 15th is just another day."

Among the minority who don't like being on salary are doctors who say they used to earn interest on the tax money they'd put aside for the quarterly tax payments; they're outvoted, however, by those who have never been able to budget properly for tax payments. Having taxes withheld in small bites out of each paycheck is "painless compared to those large quarterly payments," an Atlanta physician tells us.

Have you had any difficulty with the required corporate formalities? For example, has there been any problem with directors' meetings or the minutes? Yes, 9% No, 91%

Avoiding problems with corporate details is a matter of routine that includes keeping in touch with a lawyer. That's the consensus of respondents. In one- and two-man corporations, most indicate that they meet with their lawyer once a year, and that all the notes taken throughout the year are typed after that meeting. A Selma, Ala., solo practitioner says his lawyer makes his minutes from their telephone conversations, considering every one a meeting.

Larger groups are unable to get away with that kind of informality, though. An M.D. in a four-man group in St.

Louis says, "We've been meeting every three months since we incorporated 12 years ago."

Although the board of directors functions to satisfy the legal requirements of the corporation, survey responses show that many doctors understand that a board can be good business practice, too. As a doctor in a one-man corporation in Walla Walla, Wash., sees it: "It's a clean, orderly way to operate a medical practice." But some rank-and-file doctors in larger groups complain that their boards don't communicate with them. "We feel out of touch," is the way one Midwestern physician put it.

From your point of view, has your corporation been running smoothly? Yes, 94% No, 6%

"Things are more businesslike now," says one doctor who's representative of the overwhelming majority checking "yes" on this question. A Pittsburgh, Pa., man adds there's now a "better interaction" between the younger and the older men.

Most physicians, however, don't look upon their corporations as being anything apart from their practices. The problems and the solutions are simply carried over in their minds from self-employed practice. So, a doctor in New Hampton, N.H., writes complaining about "cash flow," and a Missouri physician says his group had problems with a man who left their corporation. In the final analysis, though, most doctors say they fall back on the advice of their lawyers, accountants, and other professionals. And the way their corporations go really depends on how good or bad that advice is.

Has your corporation been audited by the I.R.S.? Yes, 16% No, 84%

As might be expected, the I.R.S. has been dogging professional corporations with audits, but the expectation of them has apparently blunted the sting. Proof that M.D. corporations have observed prescribed procedures and, in general, kept to the straight and narrow is the fact that out of 102 audits only one reported any difficulty. And that one didn't really stem from corporate status at all.

Many respondents report that the I.R.S. didn't assess them one extra cent following audit. Even those who did have to pay more weren't really unhappy. Typical is this comment from a Chicago OBG man: "The I.R.S. was in our office at intervals over a four-month period. The only complaint we received had to do with the 100 per cent professional-car deductions we'd taken."

Not one respondent reports difficulties involving the wage-price freeze that was in effect during the years covered by the audits. Also, there are no reports of difficulties over the operation of pension and profit-sharing plans, though one doctor did have trouble with his corporation's group insurance plan. His corporation supplied more than the legally tax-free $50,000 of coverage on him, so he had to pay income tax on the premiums for the amount in excess of $50,000.

One doctor with an aggravating audit problem is in Cedar Rapids, Iowa. He incorporated just at the time the I.R.S. was questioning large deductions for overseas travel that he'd taken in previous years. He continued to travel and to deduct the cost on his corporate returns, so when the audit dragged on, it spilled over to the corporation.

At last report, his case still hasn't been settled, and he's spent thousands on legal and accounting fees to defend himself. To top it all off, his pension and profit-sharing plans have taken it on the chin in the market. "I'm sick of the whole thing," he writes.

Do you feel your advisers are giving you the service you need to run your corporation as well as possible? Yes, 80% No, 20%

Many respondents checked "no" to this question because of the bum steers they say they get from their investment advisers. But lawyers, accountants, and others come in for a share of the roasting, too. Part of the problem seems to be in communications. For example, a Drexel, N.C., doctor complains that his advisers don't pay enough attention to details, and a California surgeon adds: "I feel they're padding and extending services to increase their fees."

Another Californian feels his lawyer and accountant are too slow in responding to his problems. That theme runs through many complaints.

A 60-year-old Eugene, Ore., physician has a strong gripe about his pension plan: "It's a complicated one developed by a big insurance company. I don't understand it. My accountant doesn't understand it. My lawyer doesn't understand it. My local insurance man doesn't understand it, and the carrier's headquarters won't give any information."

An M.D. from Rockledge, Fla., complains that instead of giving advice his accountant simply does paperwork. Despite such complaints, only a few respondents report having changed advisers. One of those is a Colorado Springs man who says he's satisfied now—but only after switching advisers twice to get the service he wants.

What do you think is the best single piece of advice you've gotten to help make your corporation a success?

"Act like a corporation and be a corporation—then you don't worry." So writes a Lubbock, Tex., physician who sums up the dominant theme of respondents answering this question. That Texas doctor has proof of what he says: His eight-man group was audited by the I.R.S., and there were "no problems." A Janesville, Wis., member of a three-man corporation echoes that with, "Be honest, don't get fancy, and play the game by the rules." His group was also audited and "passed with flying colors." A frequent variation on that theme is to "keep good records" and run the professional corporation "in a businesslike manner."

Some respondents say advice on the corporate side has to be tempered with the admonition to "Think like a corporation, practice like a physician." A Yonkers, N.Y., doctor says he's been advised to "Act like a corporation for business reasons, but treat your patients like individuals."

Other nuggets of advice from respondents include: "Put your family on a budget," from a Washington, D.C., neurologist; "Have the equivalent of three or four months of income to live on while the corporation gets started;" and finally what's for many the best advice of all, "Get the best corporation specialist you can find."

What do you feel was the biggest mistake you made in your incorporating experience?

"Not doing it sooner," a Duluth, Minn., doctor replies. And he draws a lot of agreement. That's the most frequent single response to this question.

The biggest mistake one Pennsylvania doctor reports he made was "employing the wrong people to start the corporation." Attorneys, accountants, trust officers, and insurance men all get their share of listings as "biggest mistakes." A key decision in incorporating is getting the right people to help you. (For details, see Chapter 4.) If you're not satisfied, switch!

HOW MUCH SHOULD YOU EARN

"Do I earn enough to make incorporation worthwhile?" That's usually the first question that comes up when a doctor considers making the move—even though there are other possibly more important considerations he should look into. One way to answer that question is to look at the incidence of incorporation according to doctors' income levels.

Until now, there were no authoritative figures of that type, but a recent Medical Economics Continuing Survey has provided them. As you can see from the accompanying chart, if you're above the $80,000 income level, there's a clear indication incorporation is feasible for you: More than 50 per cent of doctors earning that much have already incorporated. In lower brackets, incorporation looks less feasible—especially when you get below $40,000, at which point incorporation appears to be a rarity.

You shouldn't be guided by figures alone, of course. For one thing, they measure what incorporated doctors are earning now in salary, bonus, and retirement plan contributions and not what they were earning when they decided to incorporate. And more important, income level is only part of the story.

Suppose you're a man with high income, say $100,000, but you're spending almost every penny you earn. You couldn't incorporate no matter how much you'd save in taxes— unless you could bring yourself to take the cut in current income that's required to make a significant contribution to the retirement plan.

Have you ever thought you'd be better off practicing as an unincorporated doctor again? Yes, 18% No, 82%

This question brings out many of the things that really bug incorporated doctors—the prohibition on scooping up all the money in the till if they want to, the additional expenses and extra details, and the additional reliance on

---

TO MAKE INCORPORATION PAY?

Another key question in the decision to incorporate is how much will it cost for the retirement benefits you must provide for your staff. If it's a lot, the cost could cancel out much of your tax savings. On the other hand, the corporate fringe benefits—the ones in addition to a retirement plan—may be just the dish for you.

The fact is, if you can come up with the right answers to the other questions, your income level may offer no problem even if you have only average earnings from your practice.

MOST HIGH-EARNING M.D.s ARE INCORPORATED

Doctors income level	Per cent incorporated
$90,000 or more	63%
$80,000-89,999	55
$70,000-79,999	48
$60,000-69,999	47
$50,000-59,999	33
$40,000-49,999	21
$30,000-39,999	9
Less than $30,000	4

outside advice that's required, for example.

A Brooklyn pathologist sums up the problem of being on a salary: "I can't pay large personal expenses when they come up." A Chicago man adds that he believes being self-employed again would give him more freedom. A Yonkers, N.Y., physician agrees with that, but he points out that "the financial considerations of corporate practice are overriding."

As for extra costs, increased malpractice insurance premiums and workmen's compensation costs annoy one doctor, the added expense of the extra paperwork bothers another, and the double tax on corporate profits irritates a third. Still, for most respondents, corporate tax benefits far outweigh the costs.

All things considered, are you glad you incorporated? Yes, 95% No, 5%

With 19 out of 20 incorporated doctors checking "yes" to that question, you know that incorporation has a lot going for it. You probably couldn't get that kind of affirmative response for unincorporated group practice, or even for marriage. What is it, exactly, that they like?

"Even after I put money aside for retirement, life insurance, and health benefits, I have more money than before to spend," a 52-year-old solo corporate from Knoxville, Tenn., notes. "Even at my age, the corporation will assure my retirement," a 62-year-old Californian explains.

A 51-year-old Santa Cruz, Calif., physician puts it this way: "I regret that I had to practice for 25 years without the benefits of corporation. My life and my finances would have been much better if I had fully used those 25 years."

That won't happen to a 35-year-old Jacksonville, Fla., doctor. "I incorporated the first day I went into practice," he says, "and I love it."

Many doctors indicate that they rechecked their situations after the Keogh contribution limit was raised to $7,500 a year, but they still found incorporation pays.

The one doctor who has to be given highest marks for pluck, perhaps, is the Pennsylvania man whose wife divorced him because his take-home pay dropped after incorporating. He, too, checked off "yes" to this question.

2 ARE YOU THE CORPORATE TYPE?

Incorporation may be a financial wonder drug for physicians, but there are contraindications in certain cases and if yours is one of them, incorporation could be more harmful than helpful. So, despite all you've read and heard about the advantages of incorporating your practice, better make sure you're not one of the contra-indicated types before you take the step.

From my own experience as well as other lawyers and consultants who've been instrumental in setting up professional corporations, I've found there are several kinds of doctors who should be especially cautious before reaching a decision as to whether to commit themselves to the corporate life.

Consider the man who:

Isn't sure he'll stay with the corporation. It takes time for corporate advantages like pension or profit-sharing plans to build up their big financial edge over non-corporate practice. And if you aren't sure you'll want to stay in the group you're in now, or in the one you're contemplating starting or joining, you run the risk of losing those advantages—and more. One doctor who joined an existing corporation, then left before his pension and profit-sharing benefits became his property, lost more than $29,000 in benefits and accounts receivable. Better be pretty well convinced that the group is going to be harmonious before you commit yourself to incorporation. (If you're solo, remember that you'll have to shoulder the extra incorporation costs alone.)

Spends too much. The old saying that it takes money to make money was never more apt than in describing how you benefit from a professional corporation. The corporation's contributions to your retirement fund are tax-deductible, certainly, but you still have to leave enough money in the corporation so it can make the contribution.

For example, a doctor in the 50 per cent tax bracket who put $10,000 a year into a profit-sharing fund would cut his tax bill by $5,000, but he would still have to take a $5,000 cut in his take-home pay to do it. (The $10,000 he put away, less the $5,000 tax deduction.) A doctor who's living on every penny he earns is going to feel pinched by the cut in take-home pay.

W. Fred Mangan, vice president of the professional management firm of Black and Skaggs Associates, Battle Creek, Mich., tells of one three-man group of G.P.s that has been so hard-pressed following the cut in current pay that they've been borrowing to finance current expenses. "I don't give that corporation much chance of survival," Mangan says.

Frets about the Internal Revenue Service. If you're the kind of person who gets edgy about an I.R.S. audit, you should realize that you're much more likely to get involved with the Government when you incorporate. Edward Pesin, a Newark, N.J., attorney who's formed many professional corporations, puts it this way: "Incorporation doesn't bring on an audit, but it opens up all sorts of new possibilities for questions when one actually takes place."

Therefore, you must be prepared for a much more protracted and much more difficult examination—one you probably won't be able to handle without the help of a qualified tax adviser. You're likely to be asked about how the corporation has been run, questions such as whether the board of directors has held meetings and whether the salary and other payments are proper. Then there is a whole new area the agent might explore. That's how you've set up and run the retirement plan. Those would be an addition to the routine questions about substantiating deductions and whether expenses were truly professional or whether they were personal and therefore nondeductible.

While you won't have to worry about going to court over the question of whether doctors can legally incorporate, there's always a chance that an I.R.S. agent will claim your corporation isn't operating properly. If that happens, you could still wind up with problems.

Is unwilling to attend to detail. When you incorporate, you must keep your books in apple-pie order. The I.R.S., of course, demands that. "A corporation entails more exacting record-keeping," says W. Dean Hopkins, a Cleveland attorney who successfully defended one of the professional corporation cases in the U.S. Circuit Court of Appeals. "The corporation is, legally, a separate person."

How much extra bookkeeping is involved? Marshall I. Wolper, a Miami fringe benefit specialist who's been dealing with many professional corporations, puts the increase at 10 per cent. If you can't get help with the record-keeping, then that extra load will probably fall on you. Even if you delegate the work to aides, remember, the responsibility for it is yours.

The bookkeeping work is just one part of the extra detail involved in a corporation. Other corporate affairs will demand time, too. The board of directors will have to hold meetings periodically; it has to make all policy decisions and keep a formal record of decisions on pay, coverage, vacations, days off, and other minutiae that you and your partners may have been used to settling informally.

Can't compromise on investment and retirement goals. Since the main benefits of incorporation come from the retirement plan, that's going to assume a greater and greater role in your asset accumulation. In a five-man group grossing $500,000 a year, for example, it won't be long before the retirement plan will have hundreds of thousands of dollars in it.

"A group of doctors who can't agree on their investment objectives may have special problems," says Hopkins. And Thomas H. Crawford Jr., a Jacksonville, Fla., attorney and a participant in another successful U.S. Circuit Court case, adds, "If a doctor is a wheeler-dealer with his own investments, he's going to be frustrated by having a substantial portion of his cash diverted into the retirement plan."

Another problem type is the man who is interested in squirreling away a large portion of his current income for the future. A corporation offers such a man the additional incentive of tax shelter for the money he puts aside. The problem arises when he has to mesh his goals with those of others in a group. His colleagues may be unwilling or unable to give up as much as he'd like to. (However, see Chapter 9 for some ways to solve such problems.)

Wants a lot of independence. If you like to work alone, you shouldn't combine with others just for the financial advantages you can get from incorporating. "That's like marrying for money," says Edward F. Harris, a Miami fringe benefit consultant. "If you don't want to be in a partnership, you probably won't be any happier in a corporation," he adds.

Even if you're already in a group, you may find that a corporation will leave you less independence than you have at present. Some partnerships are loosely knit, so that the partners practice pretty much as they please. You can't have that in a corporation. You must accept the management decisions of the board of directors. What's more, you may have little chance to make such decisions on your own.

Doesn't earn enough. No doubt, most doctors could gain financial advantages from a corporation, even if they have relatively low earnings. However, there are complications and extra work in forming and running a corporation. At what point do the costs outweigh the advantages? That will vary, of course, but Edward Pesin ventures a rule of thumb.

"A doctor with an annual taxable income of less than $40,000—net from all sources, less personal exemptions and deductions—will probably not gain enough from a corporation to make the extra trouble and expense worthwhile," Pesin says.

Like any rule of thumb, that may not apply in your case, but it's a good starting point. You probably shouldn't even think of incorporating if your earnings are $5,000 or more under that figure. And you should consider very carefully if they're between $35,000 and $40,000. (See the box on pages 18-19 for specific figures on doctors who've incorporated.)

On the other hand, a young doctor whose income is rising so fast that he can benefit from income averaging may find it unwise to incorporate now, even with an income well above the $40,000 figure.

The doctor with low earnings is the last of several for whom professional corporation experts deem the side effects of incorporation potentially threatening. There are doubtless many others. So a word of warning: Make sure that you really know what corporate practice will mean to you. If you have any doubts, then you should resolve them before you take the step. There's always the possibility that you just aren't the corporate type.

3 Will It Pay You to Incorporate?

With a chance to save up a tax-deductible $7,500 a year in a Keogh retirement plan, who needs to incorporate? "Hardly anyone." That, in effect, is the question and answer banks, insurance companies, brokerage firms and other institutions are pounding home these days as they jump at the selling opportunity created by the new, higher limits for the self-employed.

There's no doubt that the new ceilings of 15 per cent of professional income up to a dollar maximum of $7,500 a year allow you to save a handsome retirement fund—if you have enough working years left to do it. Paradoxically, the more you save in a Keogh fund, the more you'll be squeezed by the tax laws. One provision of those laws effectively locks in the money until you're almost 60. In fact, the prospect of the money they'll make by managing a captive retirement fund is one of the main reasons that the institutions are pushing Keogh over incorporation.

Self-interest aside, there's one thing to be said for the advertising push. It's forced many doctors to rethink the entire question of Keogh and incorporation. And even if you've already made up your mind, you may be surprised at the outcome of a fresh comparison of your situation. The case histories below provide a good starting point.

A group considering disincorporating

There's a three-man incorporated group putting away an average of $10,000 a year into their retirement plans for each man. They've been beguiled by the idea of going back to their partnership arrangement where each man drew out a share of the net profits and anything left at the end of the year was casually split up. Each man would be free to contribute to Keogh or not. At their earnings level, contributions could come to $7,500 a year per man or almost as much as they're now depositing in their corporate retirement plans.

Problem: With differing life styles and needs, the group has been troubled by the retirement program that requires all the doctors to put away the same percentage of their salaries. Last year, they tried to attract a new man, but he actually rejected their offer because he felt he would need all his income to live on for a few years and couldn't afford to put away the required retirement plan contribution.

Conclusion: Even though Keogh would allow them more flexibility on contributions and would provide them with almost as much retirement benefits, they decided to remain a corporation. What tipped the scale in their case was the extra fringe benefits they got from the corporation.

The corporation pays their families' medical and dental bills. It also pays their medical and disability insurance premiums as well as a large part of their life insurance. All those payments are tax deductible. If they had to pay them out of their own pockets, they'd have to earn about $8,000 each to come up with the after-tax dollars. So, while the law raising Keogh limits has narrowed the retirement plan gap, other standard corporate fringe benefits still tip the scale against the self-employed.

What's more, the group is contemplating some fancy leasing arrangements that will allow the doctors to transfer ownership of their practice equipment to their children. The corporation will then rent the equipment with the payments taxed at the lowest levels. When their accountant got through with his paperwork, even the doctor who'd been strapped for contributions was convinced that the extra fringe benefits made incorporation worthwhile.

A young doctor without any retirement program at all

This doctor is in his mid-30s, in practice a few years and struggling to pay back money he borrowed to complete his education, save up for a house and meet what seems like the insatiable costs of his payroll and other practice expenses. With all that, he feels he'd like to start saving money.

Problem: Because of his tight financial situation, this doctor can't put away more than $2,000 or $3,000 a year. That's well under the maximum he's allowed under Keogh, let alone the higher amount permitted under a corporate plan. (The limit on comparable corporate plans is 25 per cent of salary—equal to 20 per cent of net practice earnings—up to a maximum of $26,825 a year.) Likewise, he doesn't have an extensive insurance program, so he wouldn't get much of an advantage from the extra corporate fringe benefits.

Conclusion: Keogh is clearly the choice for this man right now. He can put the money in a savings account for a minimum cost and get the full benefit of the tax deduction. If he incorporated, the extra administrative costs of the corporation and the corporate retirement plan would eat up most of the tax savings. Incidentally, he could start a special type of plan known as an Individual Retirement Account. That will allow him to put away only $1,500 a year, but he doesn't have to contribute anything for his employes.

However, that decision should be reevaluated at frequent intervals. If that doctor follows the pattern, his earnings will approach or top the $50,000 mark in a few years. Assuming that his financial strain will ease, he'll be able to put away $7,500 a year. If he puts that away in Keogh, look what will happen:

(1) There'll be a sizeable and growing fund (about $200,000 after 15 years and well over $300,000 in 20 at present long-term bank interest) that can't be tapped for any emergency except disability or death without paying a penalty of 10 per cent in addition to the regular tax. That's what the law specifies for Keogh withdrawals before age 59½. In a corporate plan, he could borrow the money without paying any tax at all.

(2) It will be complicated or expensive to achieve investment flexibility. While the bank account will do nicely for a relatively small sum of money, financial prudence dictates that the money be spread around when the fund mounts up.

It's possible to switch Keogh investments from one place to another, say from a bank to a mutual fund, or vice versa, but it can take hours of phone calls and letters. It's also possible to get a program that allows you to switch investments without changing plans, but the administrative costs are high. Corporate plans can be structured to allow you to shift your investments with just one telephone call.

(3) Retirement planning is difficult. Assuming that the doctor got through his career without having to withdraw any money from his Keogh fund—entailing taxes and penalties—and that he was able to live with the investment restrictions, he'd have to stop working whether he wanted to or not once he reached age 70½. By that time, his fund would be approaching $1,000,000 if he put in $7,500 a year and bank interest rates held up. That large sum and the interest it generated would have to be paid out to him over the next 10 years and would create a whopping tax problem if he had practice income besides. In a corporate plan, the money doesn't have to be paid out until *you* decide to retire.

An older physician who wants to catch up

In contrast to the younger doctor, take someone in the mid-50s who's never been able to save any real money. Now the children are grown and out of college so expenses are down and, at the same time, earnings are near the peak so his income is up. He'd like to make up for lost time by accumulating as large a retirement fund as possible as fast as he can.

Problem: Despite his means and ability, the law limits the doctor if he chooses a conventional plan—$7,500 a year for Keogh and $26,825 a year for corporate. There is another kind of plan known as a defined benefit plan in which he can set a retirement payment goal and put away the amount of money he needs to reach the goal.

Conclusion: While a defined benefit Keogh plan allows far more leeway than even the increased ceiling of $7,500 on the usual type, the defined benefit corporate plan allows still more. Assuming his earnings top the $50,000 mark, the doctor could accumulate $250,000 at 65 with a defined benefit Keogh plan. Under a corporate setup, he could have a fund three times that size provided his earnings and personal finances permit it. To reach that higher corporate goal, he'd have to net about $125,000 a year and be able to put away $50,000.

What it comes down to is that an older man can put away as much under a corporate setup as he can afford to and catch up with a younger man who's been putting the money away all along. That's not recommended, of course, because unless you put away the money year-by-year, you may not be able to make the contributions required for a high-powered program later on. However, if you're in the same boat as the man here, you have to do something and the corporate plan is probably the thing to do.

One more consideration that's especially important for the older doctor is the advantage that corporate retirement funds have over Keogh if he should die before he gets to draw out the money for his retirement. The corporate retirement plan is exempt from Federal estate tax, so there'd be more for his family.

The financially addled doctor

You know this man. He works hard and plays hard and never finds time to meet with his tax adviser. His quarterly tax payments are late and he usually ends up owing money on his tax return even after it's filed. While he earns a lot, he always seems to be behind.

Problem: The last thing this doctor needs is to be harnessed to a corporation. He'd have to take his pay on a regular basis as salary and make the tax payments on time—possibly every time he's paid. And not only would he have to listen to his accountant, he'd also have to meet with a lawyer and possibly even an actuary.

Conclusion: With all those problems, it would be almost impossible to incorporate such a doctor's practice and make it work. Casual financial habits led one jury to a decision that broke up a professional corporation. Even if this man got into court, the rigid deadlines and disciplines of corporate life would probably be too much for him.

While his income would permit the doctor to put away the maximum $7,500 a year in Keogh, he probably wouldn't be able to do that every year. Still, it would be worthwhile to start the retirement program. If anything, there would be an advantage to the Keogh tax lock-in feature for this doctor—he'd be less tempted to tamper with the retirement money for frivolous purposes.

A high-earning doctor

With four out of 10 physicians in private practice earning $60,000 or more, according to a recent Medical Economics survey, there are plenty in this situation. Take a man in his mid-40s earning about $70,000 who's putting away the maximum allowable $7,500 a year in a Keogh plan. He's worried about his income tax bill that's uncomfortably close to the $20,000 mark and he'd like to put away more than Keogh permits.

Problem: Even though he knows that if he incorporated

INCORPORATION OR NOT—AT A GLANCE

Despite the Pension Reform Act of 1974 which attempted to narrow the difference between Keogh and corporate retirement plans, incorporation still has a decided edge if you've got the money to make it worthwhile and if you're going to be comfortable practicing in that setup. The chart below will help you pinpoint the differences.

	UNINCORPORATED	INCORPORATED
Retirement plans	Usual type of Keogh allows maximum deduction of 15% of net up to $7,500 a year annually.	Comparable plan allows maximum deduction of 20% of net income (25% of corporate salary) up to maximum of $26,825* a year annually.
	Defined benefit plan allows accumulation of fund to provide retirement payment of $50;000 a year.	Comparable plan allows accumulation of fund to provide retirement payment of $80,475* a year.
	Contributions for staff employes must be at same percentage as for doctors and money belongs to them immediately.	Contributions for staff can be at lower percentage because Social Security can be counted toward payments and ownership can be postponed by postponing vesting.
	Investment flexibility can be achieved at a cost.	Complete investment discretion can be provided.

	UNINCORPORATED	INCORPORATED
	Tax laws exact a penalty for payments before age 59½ and require payout beginning at age 70½.	No restriction on payouts.
	Additional contributions out of after-tax income limited to 10% of income, but a maximum of $2,500 a year and permitted only if there are any office employes participating.	Only restrictions on additional contributions are percentage limits—effectively 6% of salary in most cases, but up to 10% allowed.
	No estate tax benefits.	Amounts not drawn for retirement exempt from Federal estate tax.
Additional fringe benefits	Not available.	Tax deductible payments for life, medical and disability insurance and for medical and dental bills.
Income	Simplified bookkeeping; taxed as collected.	Sophisticated reporting and can be split to achieve lowest rates.
Expenses	Lower practice costs, but higher retirement plan fees unless money is invested in savings bank.	Higher legal and accounting fees.

*To be raised to keep pace with inflation.

and went on a salary he could increase his retirement plan contributions to 25 per cent of the salary (equal to 20 per cent of his current, unincorporated net), the doctor is concerned about what it would cost him to cover his employes. He has a large staff and they're satisfied with Keogh.

Conclusion: This doctor is an ideal candidate for incorporation. Not only would he have the benefit of the increased retirement plan contributions, he could also have the advantage of the other tax deductible corporate fringe benefits. Assuming that the additional fringe benefits came to about $4,000 and that he had an additional $1,000 in extra corporate expenses, the doctor would have $65,000 left to divide between his salary and retirement program. On a salary of $52,000, he'd be able to put away $13,000 or $5,500 more than he could under Keogh.

So, counting all the fringe benefits, the $70,000-a-year doctor would reduce his taxable income by $9,500 if he incorporates at a tax-deductible cost of $1,000. What about the problem of covering the employes? Actually, there wouldn't be any. The corporate arrangement would allow him to credit part of the money he pays for Social Security toward the corporate contributions—known as "integration"—so right off, he'd reduce the amount for his employes to about 20 per cent.

While the initial cost would be somewhat higher than the Keogh plan, in the long run it probably wouldn't be much more and could be actually lower. How's that? Simply through the forfeitures that the employes would leave behind if they left before they got full ownership of the amounts in their accounts. The forfeited amounts would be credited to the corporation's contributions. In Keogh, once a contribution is made, it belongs to the employe forever.

A doctor involved in a major career change

Take someone who's been working in a group who's now going to strike out on his own. That's for illustrative purposes, it could be someone who's planning to switch locations or type of practice. Anyway, this doctor now has a high

---

BUILDING UP A RETIREMENT FUND

As you can see from the figures below, you can accumulate a sizable retirement nest egg in a corporate retirement plan. While the money will be subject to income tax when it's withdrawn (but it's exempt from Federal estate tax if you die first), your fund will still provide a handsome retirement income if you save consistently for a number of years.

Nest egg if you put away $15,000 a year and the number of years to retirement is . . .*

		10	15	20	25	30
. . . and the fund earns	6%	$198,983	$352,790	$559,942	$ 838,947	$1,214,727
	7½	214,366	398,319	665,836	1,051,767	1,612,504
	9	231,275	451,230	794,476	1,330,110	2,165,971

Nest egg if you put away $25,000 a year and the number of years to retirement is . . .*

		10	15	20	25	30
. . . and the fund earns	6%	$331,639	$587,982	$ 933,237	$1,398,245	$2,024,544
	7½	357,276	663,864	1,108,393	1,752,945	2,687,507
	9	385,458	752,049	1,324,126	2,216,849	3,609,949

**Assuming deposits are made at the end of each year and that interest is compounded quarterly.*

income and good prospects even after the change.

Problem: Even though the prospects of continued high income may be good, there's always a risk associated with a change. Besides, even though the receipts may be high, the startup expenses involved in a new practice might eat up all the profits.

Conclusion: Unless the doctor is already incorporated, it appears that he should wait and see how things go for a couple of years before taking the step. Meanwhile, he can put away whatever he can afford in a Keogh plan so that he doesn't break his stride on his retirement planning.

One caution: If the doctor's already incorporated, it wouldn't make sense to break it up just because of the career change. The startup expenses have already been paid and there would be additional fees associated with a termination. Until he gets his bearings, the doctor could keep the fringe benefit programs down to a minimum. When he can again afford it, reactivating them will be a simple matter.

As you can see, even though Keogh is now closer to corporation retirement plans, the unincorporated doctor is still at a disadvantage. Despite that, incorporation isn't the answer for everyone. You'll have to work out the figures with your adviser, but before that you can get a rough idea of where you stand by doing the same kind of analysis as was done in this article. Remember, when you're comparing your own situation, consider how much money the law and your finances allow you to put away and how much you can benefit from the additional fringe benefits available to corporations. If both are limited, then you should consider Keogh.

4 | You Need Specialist Help to Incorporate

The Internal Revenue Service may have lost its war against professional corporations, but don't expect complete capitulation without prolonged guerilla skirmishes. The I.R.S. has declared that it will continue to judge medical corporations on a case-by-case basis, looking for imperfections in the corporate structure and for situations that don't jibe with state law or court decisions. It it does find such flaws, it could seek to have the corporation declared invalid.

To counter that line of attack, doctors planning to incorporate will need the best legal and business advice they can get. "Instead of going after professional corporations on principle," predicts a New Jersey lawyer who has set up numerous medical corporations, "the I.R.S. will go after the individual corporations it feels are most loosely formed and sloppiest in their record-keeping. There's always the danger that a court may disallow a particular corporation for not following proper procedures, but now that the courts have laid out the ground rules, the danger can be avoided. It's a case of making sure everyone concerned with forming and running the corporation faces the facts and does his homework."

One fact a doctor will have to face early in his incorporation planning is this: The attorney and the accountant who regularly handle his affairs may not be qualified to deal with the complexities of incorporation in a manner that will turn aside I.R.S. attacks. So the doctor must be willing to do in his business affairs exactly what he does in his practice: call in well-qualified specialists. An attorney who is an expert on professional incorporation is a must. The doctor may decide he also needs the services of an actuary. His accountant, management consultant, and insurance adviser all should take a hand.

Impartial advice is vital at this stage, so the would-be incorporator must be sure the expert isn't selling anything besides advice. In seeking a preliminary actuarial study, for example, he'd be wise to consult an independent actuary, not one connected with an underwriting firm bent on funding the doctor's retirement plan with insurance.

"The worst threat a doctor faces in incorporating now is that he'll get bad advice," says one consultant. "When a doctor incorporates, there are products and services to be sold. Many a salesman, whether he handles insurance, mutual funds, or stationery, is after his share. The doctor naturally seeks advice from people he's dealt with satisfactorily in the past. But because of the complex legal entity involved, he may wind up with expenses, legal knots, and tax problems that he never bargained for.

"I know a doctor who lost thousands of dollars in Keogh

benefits by staying out of the program on the advice of his regular accountant, who didn't understand the plan. We've run into the same thing with incorporation. Because incorporation is a very special area, some doctors will have to be prepared to work for a short period of time without the services of the very people they've come to depend on."

That warning is echoed by Clayton L. Scroggins, Cincinnati management consultant with long experience in the professional corporation field: "I know a case where a lawyer told six incorporating anesthesiologists it was all right to include a urologist who had no connection with them except that he rented space in their building. Such a setup would be an open invitation to the I.R.S. to contend that this was a corporation existing only to avoid taxes."

Assuming you decide to call in outside specialists to help your regular advisers set up the corporation, be prepared for the possibility of some friction. Specialization isn't as fully accepted in the legal and accounting fields as it is in medicine, and your long-time attorney or accountant may be reluctant to accept the advice of an outsider, no matter what his qualifications.

"I walk on eggs to help the doctor maintain his relationship with his old advisers," one attorney explains. "I may be able to set up a corporation, but the local attorney or accountant who knows details of the doctor's separation agreement with his first wife or his private real-estate holdings is very important to the doctor's day-to-day handling of affairs."

Finding suitable advisers is an imprecise art hinging on such variables as geography (almost all the men acknowledged by their peers to be expert in the field are located in metropolitan areas), your own personal reaction to a man and his views, and the time you can devote to checking out the candidates. Before talking to any of them, spend some time acquainting yourself with incorporation features and terminology. Learn the difference between pension and profit sharing and what's meant by vesting, for example, so that you'll be in a better position to judge the person's answers.

Once you find one specialist for your team, the rest may fall in place through cross references. The attorney, for example, may be able to direct you to a specializing C.P.A., or the actuary may be able to recommend a competent attorney.

A reputable medical management consultant firm with some experience in incorporation may be the best over-all solution. Such a firm can do a preliminary study to determine if incorporation is feasible for you. If the answer is Yes, the consultant can undoubtedly recommend experienced men in your area. To find management consultant firms, check with the Society of Professional Business Consultants (221 North LaSalle Street, Chicago, Ill. 60601) and your state medical society, then talk to colleagues. Once you have a candidate, ask him about his background in incorporation work and for references from medical groups he's incorporated or done studies for.

If you set out to find your own advisers, a capable attorney should be your major concern. Sound legal advice is the cornerstone on which to build a strong medical corporation. Check out a likely candidate in three general areas:

1. The attorney needs a strong background in pension and profit-sharing plans. Such plans represent the greatest tax loss for the Government and therefore will be given the sharpest scrutiny by the I.R.S.

"Pension and profit-sharing plans can get terribly complex," says Michael H. Rotman, a Chicago attorney who has worked with numerous medical corporations. "You have to know the strengths and weaknesses of each type of plan and decide which is best for a particular group of doctors or if a combination of the two is needed. And there are matters of discrimination in vesting, integrating with Social Security, and administering the plan. Retirement planning is a field by itself, and the big income gaps between professional and nonprofessional employes in a medical corporation complicate matters further."

An attorney's unfamiliarity with pension and profit-sharing plans could have unfortunate results, according to Roger Harrison, Norman, Okla., management consultant. "We've found attorneys setting up retirement programs by filling in the blanks on how-to-do-it forms provided by insurance companies," he says. "That's a pretty dangerous way of going about it in view of the sums of money involved and the potential I.R.S. scrutiny."

2. The attorney needs specific knowledge of professional corporations. "There are special problems a lawyer won't know about unless he's dealt with medical groups," warns Jule M. Hannaford, a Minneapolis attorney who has handled hundreds of professional corporations and serves as counsel for the Medical Group Management Association and the Minnesota State Medical Association. "For example, a lawyer normally tries to give a corporation as much flexibility as possible and leave decisions to the board of directors. But I find that doctors want all the details, such as days off and vacations, spelled out in the incorporation documents."

"Each state's enabling legislation for professional corporations is different," Michael Rotman adds, "and with the scrutiny we expect these corporations to get from the I.R.S., it's important that the enabling act be followed to the letter."

3. The attorney should be familiar with I.R.S. procedures and policies in the district where the corporation will be based. "It's always an advantage in tax matters to have an attorney who has worked with district officials, but there's a special reason in medical incorporation," Rotman points out. "Each district has its own interpretation of the various rules on how to set up a retirement program. Normally, an attorney files a corporate plan with the I.R.S., and if there are objections the attorney and the I.R.S. can work it out and amend the plan. However, an attorney who knows local district interpretations can save a doctor considerable trouble and may even prevent his losing his deduction by drawing up a plan that meets district requirements without the need for involved amendments."

Finding an attorney who meets these general requirements may take some shopping around. Of course, if your regular attorney knows a specialist in the field and can work with him, your problems are solved. If he doesn't, cross-check several sources for names. Ask independent actuaries for the names of attorneys they find competent in dealing with professional corporations. Contact groups already incorporated and see who handled their work. Get the advice of your state medical society, the trust department of your bank, and management consultants.

If two or more sources give you the same name, you have a likely candidate. As with choosing a management consultant, ask about his previous medical incorporation work and arrange to talk to members of corporations he's set up. And talk to at least one other attorney who's been recommended. In other words, shop not for price, but for competence.

Especially good prospects are likely to be members of law firms that have long emphasized work in profit sharing and pensions and that have worked with several professional corporations in recent years.

Once you find your lawyer, he'll probably be able to help you select any other special advisers, such as an accountant. Corporate accounting and bookkeeping mechanics are fairly close to those of a partnership, although more detailed record-keeping is involved. If your regular accountant is inexperienced with corporate books, you'll need either a C.P.A. who's familiar with medical corporations and their special tax problems or a management consultant who has a strong accounting background to help set up the books. Record-keeping is a big part of maintaining the corporate structure for I.R.S. purposes, and the corporate C.P.A. may be able to give you some streamlining suggestions to ease the burden of added volume.

Experts differ on the need for an actuarial study. Attorneys Hannaford and Rotman, on the one hand, say that a doctor will benefit from spending $500 or so to have an independent actuary study the possibilities and make recommendations about his retirement needs, and funding. This helps minimize one of the traps doctors often fall into when incorporating: putting more money into retirement programs than they'll ultimately need and cutting current income dangerously short. Actuaries who specialize in this type of work can be found in most major cities. For most doctors, though, the only practical retirement plan is one in which the contributions are based on a simple percentage formula. The only limitations on such plans are the legal ceilings and the individual doctor's finances. In such cases, an actuary isn't really needed.

THIS PROFESSIONAL CORPORATION DIDN'T STAND UP

Once a professional corporation is formed, it must "make rabbit tracks in the snow from the hutch to the cornfield and back, so that if anyone ever comes to check, he will find the tracks." Those colorful words of caution are among the first that Harry V. Lamon Jr., veteran of the incorporation court battles with the I.R.S., gives when forming a professional corporation. The Atlanta lawyer had occasion to repeat that warning in a letter to the professional corporations he helped form.

The occasion was a U.S. Tax Court decision against four Wisconsin radiologists who claimed corporate tax treatment. The case, Jerome J. Roubik et al. v. Commissioner, is one of the most important cases since professionals won the right to incorporate, says Lamon. It shows that the I.R.S. and the Tax Court are, indeed, going to keep a keen eye out for corporate rabbit tracks, and it indicates what kind of tracks have to be there.

The I.R.S. finally ended its struggle to keep professional groups from being recognized as legitimate corporations under any circumstances. But in its announcement of concession, the revenue service reserved the right—in special circumstances—to challenge the tax status of income earned by the members of incorporated groups. The Roubik case was such a special circumstance.

The four radiologists incorporated under Wisconsin law in 1961, but they continued to operate their practices in just about the same way as they had before. They just consolidated their bookkeeping and opened a corporation bank account.

Each doctor, however, had a separate account under the corporation name, and at the end of a month, each drew income out of his account based on his productivity. The only expenses paid with corporation checks were contributions to a retirement plan and the cost of bookkeeping. Everything else—rent, office supplies, nurses, equipment—was paid for by the individual doctors. Each physician continued to use his own individual bill form and letterhead. And each continued to practice independently, with no corporate authority making assignments or exerting control over the quality of his work.

Under those circumstances, the court decided, the individual physicians—not the corporation—earned the income, and therefore corporate tax treatment didn't apply. "The taxpayers in this case," the decision concluded, "did not put flesh on the bones of the corporate skeleton, irrespective of the question of its legal existence under local law; thus it never became operative in any meaningful sense."

The issue in the case isn't whether the group should be classified and taxed as a corporation on the one hand or a partnership on the other, comments the tax service, U.S. Tax Week. "Rather, the issue is whether the business was actually carried on by the corporation through its employes as employes or whether it was carried on by the doctors as individuals. Certainly, at the least, the case indicates that extremely careful following of corporate procedures must be adhered to by professional service corporations." Bank accounts, for example, should be in the corporate name, the service notes, and billing should be done by the corporation.

Lawyer Lamon adds some other requirements of corporate form that, if followed, might have led to a different decision in this case. Not only should there have been just one corporate checking account, but all expenses should have been paid out of it. The doctors should have been paid salaries, rather than distributions based on productivity. The corporation should have held itself out to the public as the employer of the doctors. Each doctor should have had payments for his services by the hospitals made to the corporation in its name.

In his letter to corporate clients, Lamon advises: "By all means, hold your monthly board of governors meetings; record the minutes of those meetings; have all significant decisions made by your board of governors; and make sure that all contracts are signed by the appropriate officers of the association and the association seal affixed. In short, to be *taxed* like a corporation, you must *act* like a corporation. Substance must be more important than form."

Once you've decided on the man or men you want to set up your corporation, don't then settle for second best just because your choice isn't immediately available. Interest in professional incorporation is at an all-time high, and many specialists are swamped with inquiries. But considering the complexities of incorporating and the amount of money involved in fringe benefits, waiting for the man you want

---

AN INCORPORATED DOCTOR'S $95,350 MISTAKE

In still another successful attack on a professional corporation, a U.S. Court of Appeals upheld an extra tax assessment of $95,350.83 that the I.R.S. had levied on an Oconomowoc, Wis., surgeon. The decision wasn't just a defeat for the doctor involved; elements in the trial have ominous implications for every incorporated doctor—possibly even for unincorporated doctors.

Dr. Dean P. Epperson was working a backbreaking pace of 80 to 90 hours a week at the time his corporation was formed in 1962. Mistakenly, he paid little if any attention to the formalities. He never changed his shingle, letterheads, or bills; he held no meetings with the two other directors on the board of his corporation; worst of all, he treated the corporate funds as his own.

"The corporation never established its own bank account but placed all gross receipts of the medical practice into the taxpayer's own business account," the Government stated later in its brief to the Court of Appeals. As a result, when Epperson was audited, the I.R.S. charged that all the money he'd earned should be taxed to him as dividends from his corporation. He paid the taxes and then sued for a refund.

At the trial before a jury in U.S. District Court, the Government supplemented the dividend argument and pushed for the tax assessment on the basis that the doctor had behaved as an unincorporated practitioner, and that Epperson, rather than his

may be well worthwhile. The same holds true for fees. The specialist may charge more, but his services are likely to be well worth it.

Putting together a medical corporation that can withstand I.R.S. probes is now a fairly routine project. It's a matter of seeking the best advice available—and then following it.

---

corporation, was the "true earner of the income." Dr. Epperson appealed, but the Appeals Court upheld that decision.

The facts of the case confirm one of the key points that all incorporated physicians must consider whenever they make important practice decisions: Failing to observe the corporate amenities may well bring on expensive trouble.

But there's an added lesson in this case: Doctors in tax trouble might come in for personal attack that has little to do with tax technicalities. The Government's attorney closed his case with an impassioned speech: "We say he (Epperson) is not entitled to a refund of taxes because he hasn't paid his fair share . . . Let's make this doctor pay the kind of income taxes he ought to pay . . . I am sick and tired, and I know you are, at having to pay taxes at a (high) rate when these rich people like to construe and set up all these transactions to save taxes so they don't have to pay any."

Epperson's attorney objected to the inflammatory language but got little help from the judge, who allowed the remarks to stand even though they were "a little personal." The judges in the Appeals Court considered the statements more thoroughly and said: "We believe the quoted portions were in bad taste if not reprehensible. But . . . we have concluded that there was no prejudicial error . . . the defendant was not denied a fair trial in view of the record as a whole."

So much for the record. What will never be known is how much the let's-sock-it-to-the-rich-doctor argument influenced the jury. It took them only a half hour to find that the doctor had to pay the full $95,350.83.

5 How much will it cost to organize?

Doctors seeking to incorporate their practices have been confused to discover that legal fees for the job seem to run anywhere from a few hundred dollars to several thousand. Why should this be? For one thing, like doctors, no two lawyers work alike. For another, some lawyers are willing to cut rates in the hope of getting you as a client. What's more, some opportunists charge too much, and some well-meaning attorneys underestimate what's required and charge too little. Newcomers to the field have sometimes resorted to phoning other lawyers before quoting fees.

Even experienced men, at first quote, seem hard to pin down. Some ask a flat fee for incorporating you; others charge step-by-step with an extra hourly fee for consultations. Some include items like filing fees or a legal checkup at the end of the first year; others charge extra for them. Many do not charge for preliminary discussions; others toss them in if you buy the full incorporation package, but bill you separately if you change your mind about incorporating or switch to another attorney.

Faced with all this, how can an interested doctor decide whose price is right? The chart on page 61 will help you answer that question. It's based on estimates provided by more than a dozen leading professional-incorporation attorneys. Some of them fought key court cases in which doctors won the right to incorporate, and some were instrumental in persuading their state legislatures to legalize professional corporations. Allowing for possible geographical variations, it represents what a typical doctor should expect to pay for qualified advice and a quality job of incorporation.

"Qualified" and "quality" are key words. The man who is inexperienced in the specific area of professional medical corporations may, with the best of intentions, cost you more than you bargain for. He may, for instance, rely on "master" plans or forms drawn up to meet routine incorporation problems. Most attorneys use such forms where they apply. But the chances are your incorporation will not be a routine affair and, as attorney Richard G. Maloney of Boston points out, "It takes an experienced man to know which forms fit your situation and which forms should either be adapted or discarded entirely in favor of a tailor-made program."

"You're trying to protect thousands of dollars in potential tax savings that will be available to you down through the years under corporate pension and profit-sharing plans and other fringe benefits," says attorney Berrien C. Eaton Jr. of Phoenix. "To save a few dollars in fees, but risk having a future Internal Revenue Service challenge wipe out all those tax savings, can only be described as penny-wise and pound-foolish."

Essentially, attorneys' fees are based on hourly rates. A fee that's below the range indicated on the chart may be a bargain, but it may also cover an incomplete job. "Sure," says Edward Pesin of Newark, N.J., "I can go through the formality of incorporating a doctor for a relatively small fee. But what has he got till he sets up an I.R.S.-approved pension or profit-sharing plan? That takes hours to discuss and prepare. No lawyer can do it properly for a simple incorporation fee. Time is a lawyer's stock in trade, and a fee that seems low may simply not allow for the hours the lawyer should put into the job to do it right."

A fee that seems low may also mask a booby trap for the I.R.S. to spring later. "Newcomers to this field don't realize how difficult it is to stay ahead of the Government," says Thomas H. Crawford Jr., an attorney who practices in Jacksonville, Fla. "Not only must I be aware of the pitfalls we've successfully skirted in the past, for instance, but I have to do a lot of studying for the future. Already I've discerned a pattern of challenges likely to come up, based on claims of unreasonable compensation and dividend payouts. By planning how to avoid such problems today, we can keep a lot of doctors out of court tomorrow."

On the other end of the scale, a fee above the chart range may not be exorbitant; it may simply reflect the number of hours necessary to handle a particularly complex job. A Los Angeles attorney recalls one that involved several doctors, some more productive than others, who not only had a group practice to consider but operated a multiphasic testing-device service, too.

"We had the usual time-consuming problem of working out arrangements satisfactory to each doctor's individual financial situation. And we had to set it up so the testing operation didn't violate California's ethical standards. On top of everything else, there was a fuzzy malpractice insurance setup that had to be straightened out."

With all that in mind, here's how to use the chart:

Start with the line labeled "basic range" and go across to the column covering the number of doctors involved in your prospective corporation. (The text accompanying the chart explains what allowances you should make if more than four M.D.-stockholders are involved.) Subtract the fee for the accountant; most attorneys insist he be part of the proceedings, but getting him and paying him is your responsibility and not part of the legal fee. Add a reasonable amount for travel expenses or long-distance phone calls if you practice in an area where you can't locate qualified advice close to home.

Note that the biggest jumps are between a solo incorporation and a two-man job. As Marvin Kamensky, a Chicago attorney, explains it: "You've got to add all the extra time involved in explaining the law, and the options it allows, to two or more doctors and their advisers. The doctors may have different needs to be met by incorporation—retirement income, say, vs. current income. One may be going to retire in five years, another may still be paying off his share of the practice. Reconciling all these points of view takes time you don't need to spend on a solo corporation. A good way to cut costs here is for the doctors and their advisers to get together and iron out some of these differences before they come in to see me."

Kamensky, incidentally, believes an employment contract should be drawn up for every professional corporation. Every multi-man corporation should also have a buy-sell agreement. He feels they're needed for tax and other legal purposes. Other attorneys see little reason to include an employment contract in a solo corporation, except to give it more credibility in the eyes of the I.R.S., but they all advise it for a multiple corporation. Some charge extra for it, others simply lump it into the part of their fee allocated to the buy-sell agreement.

"It's usually almost as easy to reconcile four men as it is to work things out for two," adds Robert Pierce of Boston. "That's why fees don't jump so dramatically after you pass the first couple of levels. Of course, if working things out does get sticky, the fee will rise accordingly."

"Most incorporation attorneys will be happy to supply a list of things the doctors should try to agree upon before we come into the picture," according to Converse Murdoch, a Wilmington, Del. attorney. "That often helps to cut costs," says attorney Stanley L. Drexler of Denver, Colo.: "The doctor should keep in mind that the more doctors there are, the more portions the fee will be divided into. Despite the additional work on the attorney's part, a multiple-incorporation job for doctors who've done their homework in advance will probably cost less, per doctor, than a solo incorporation would."

Now, let's assume you're planning a solo corporation and are trying to decide between Attorneys A, B, and C, each of whom comes well recommended and seems to understand the special problems of a professional medical corporation. Attorney A says he'll do the job for $500; Attorney B for $1,400; Attorney C for $1,700.

The chart tells you the range of basic *legal* fees for forming a solo corporation is usually between $1,600 to $2,700. So you ask Attorney A what you'll be getting for $500. It turns out he's just going to incorporate you for $450 and add $50 for the out-of-pocket costs involved.

So far, a reasonable fee for an incomplete job. But now it begins to pile up. First, you'll have to pay an additional $100 for stock certificates, minute books, and a corporate seal. Next, Attorney A believes in waiting a year to set up a pension plan. When you're ready, that will cost you $1,000 more—$250 for consultations to explain your various options and to get the proper financial figures from your accountant, and a flat $750 for the plan itself. So the actual basic fee for Attorney A is not $500 but $1,600.

Attorney B's $1,400 fee, you discover, includes the orientation session, the actual incorporation, and a simple pension plan. But you'll pay all the $150 out-of-pocket and corporate-kit expenses outlined above. And if your pension plan turns out to be complicated, the additional work involved will come to $50 an hour. If it takes just four hours, Attorney B's fee for basic services will be $1,750.

Attorney C's rate, however, includes the works—orientation, incorporation, pension plan, and all out-of-pocket expenses. His $1,700 quote, originally the highest of the three, is actually giving you more for your money.

A glance at the lower portion of the chart—the optionals—will show that Attorney C's fee becomes even more reasonable. Your corporation, like any newborn baby, is going to need first-year care and a first-birthday checkup. To avoid unfavorable attention from the I.R.S., a corporation must act like one. It must put its corporate name on the door, write all correspondence on corporate letterheads, bill in the corporate name, keep proper corporate books and minutes, and observe a dozen other seemingly trivial formalities which, if not followed, could cost you your corporate tax status. (See box on page 70.)

Your own attorney and accountant can do the "policing," especially if properly prepared for it by the incorporating attorney. (William G. O'Neill of Philadelphia and George E. Ray of Dallas are typical of several attorneys who will provide checklists of things to watch out for during that first year.) But whoever does it, it's going to cost you money.

If you want Attorney A to do it, he'll charge you $50 a month as a retainer ($600 a year), including preparing the annual minutes at the end of the year. That raises his total price to $2,200. Attorney B's fees are $150 for the year-end minutes and checkup, and $50 an hour for any calls you or your advisers make upon him during the year—estimate: another $200. That raises his total fee to $2,100. But Attorney C, who likes to finish what he starts, includes that first year in his original $1,700, so long as you don't make an unreasonable number of demands upon him.

How can Attorney C afford to include this optional item in his basic fee? Because he, like many other experienced men in the field of professional incorporation, has found that the first-year checkup, except perhaps for the preparation of the minutes of the annual meeting, can be fairly routine stuff.

Now let's take a look at the other optional items that are on the chart.

Besides your own attorney's fee and the first-year checkup, there's the cost of an actuary or insurance adviser to help you set up and operate a defined-benefit pension plan. If you decide you don't want such a plan, you probably won't need this type of advice at all. And in any case, before hiring such an expert, it will pay you to consult insurance companies which are soliciting retirement-fund business or have already sold you a substantial personal policy. Many of them have departments which will do feasibility studies, and even detailed actuarial work, free—in an effort to land the account.

As for the remaining option—a second service corporation or a partnership to include your real estate and equipment, attorneys disagree on whether it's advisable or not.

A few don't believe the benefits match the disadvantages of extra expense, extra problems of administration, and an extra target for the I.R.S. to attack. But Harry V. Lamon Jr. of Atlanta, who has set up service corporations, feels that they frequently can be used to provide greater flexibility and additional financial gains.

"Nonmedical people, such as your family or friends, can own stock in such a corporation," he points out. "In a professional medical corporation, they can't. It's one way of passing some of your income along at lower tax rates. There's also the problem of the doctor who owns an interest in the building in which his incorporated group operates. He may be planning to retire someday on the income from that. He can't do it if the practice corporation owns it because, once he retires, he has to get out of that corporation. There are other factors involved, too—perhaps a trust or partnership will have more advantages than a second corporation."

The same should be said, once again, about the chart. It represents an attempt to bring order into a field of confusion, but it isn't a bible. Once you've found the adviser you want, don't quibble about slight variations—any more than you'd ask one surgeon, say, to match another's fee. Ask to have a fee explained or itemized, yes. But considering the potential tax savings involved and the fact that attorneys' and consultants' fees are tax-deductible, how much you pay for incorporation isn't nearly as important as how good a corporation you get.

A GUIDELINE TO INCORPORATION COSTS

To use the chart, first find the basic price range that applies to you. (For groups of more than four doctors, an extra $250 per man for basic expenses is a reasonable, but by no means absolute, guide.) Then add the cost of any appropriate optional services. When an attorney quotes you a fee, particularly if it's outside the range, ask him to explain what services it includes and any variation. But keep in mind that, in the long run, the best advice will usually pay for itself.

	Expense	**Solo practice**	**2-man practice**	**3- or 4-man practice**
Basic	INCORPORATION ATTORNEY			
Basic	Orientation	$200- 250	$250- 350	$350- 500
Basic	Incorporation, bylaws, and minutes	200- 500	300- 500	350- 500
Basic	Pension or profit-sharing plan	750-1,000	850-1,200	950-1,200
Basic	Disability insurance and medical reimbursement plan	100- 200	100- 200	100- 200
Basic	Employment contract and buy-sell agreement	Usually unnecessary	300- 500	350- 600
Basic	OUT-OF-POCKET EXPENSES			
Basic	Filing fees, stock certificates, minute books, corporate seal	100- 250	100- 250	100- 250
Basic	Accountant	250- 500	250- 600	250- 600
Basic	**Basic range**	**$1,600-3,700**	**$2,150-3,600**	**$2,450-3,850**
Optional	Personal attorney or business consultant	$250- 500	$250- 600	$250- 750
Optional	Actuary or insurance consultant	0- 500	0- 500	0- 500
Optional	Additional pension plan	500- 750	600-1,000	600-1,000
Optional	First-year checkup	200- 600	200- 600	200- 600
Optional	**Optional range**	**$950-2,350**	**$1,050-2,700**	**$1,050-2,850**
	Total range	**$2,550-5,050**	**$3,200-6,300**	**$3,600-6,700**

6 | INCORPORATION: THE FIRST KEY STEPS

Changing your practice into a corporation resembles the metamorphosis of a caterpillar into a butterfly—a lawyer takes your earthbound organization and a few weeks later it flies away as a corporation.

While it's true that, like the caterpillar, you don't control each step of the change, it's equally true that your small part is vital to the ultimate success of the venture. Your most important role will be to supply the financial data that your attorney and other advisers need to plan the corporation. You'll also have to make the important decisions on how much to put aside for fringe benefits and how your corporation will be organized. The more informed you are, the better your decisions will be.

Experienced attorneys operate from that premise, and they consequently spend a lot of time explaining what's happening to clients who want to form professional corporations. Three attorneys who have formed hundreds of professional corporations repeated those explanations. What they told me jibes with my experience in forming professional corporations.

Two of the attorneys are Thomas H. Crawford Jr., of Jacksonville, Fla., and Harry V. Lamon Jr., of Atlanta, each of whom participated in one of the United States Circuit Court of Appeals decisions that ultimately forced the I.R.S. to give up its opposition to professional corporations. The third is Edward Pesin, of Newark, N.J., who helped push through his state's professional corporation act.

While the specific steps of the incorporation process will vary according to the style of the attorney you select, the needs of your organization, and the laws of your state, these three men follow a seven-step incorporation procedure.

Before you take any of those steps, though, there are several you'll want to take on your own. First, of course, you'll have to decide whether you're even interested in incorporating. That may require some discussion with your wife and your colleagues to make sure you're in agreement on the need to save for retirement. Then you'll have to find a well-qualified lawyer. Finally, you should ask him how much it's going to cost you to incorporate. Perhaps you won't get a precise figure, but you should get minimum and maximum costs. (For some information on the costs, see previous chapter.)

After you've attended to those preliminaries, you'll be ready to take the seven basic steps:

Choosing the fringe benefits. This is probably the most important single step of all, since it's the one that will give you the best measure of your potential tax savings—the main goal of incorporation. Your retirement plan, the biggest single fringe, will probably be a major topic of your first meeting with your lawyer, but you needn't make the final choice of any benefits until after you've completed the other steps. (See Chapter 8 for details on retirement plans.) Even after you decide on what fringe benefits you want and the level of payments you'll make, you can always change your mind—but, in some situations, it may cost you extra money to get the revisions. So it's important to choose carefully. Crawford explains the various types of plans and how the assets of each will fit into the incorporators' estate-building plans. He says that incorporation frequently necessitates revamping a doctor's estate plan.

Lamon discusses retirement plans by contrasting the way a doctor's assets will build up in a corporation with the prospect if he doesn't incorporate. To prepare for that briefing, Lamon has his doctor-clients fill out detailed questionnaires about their earnings and expenses, including the salaries of employes.

Just that kind of information is one of the most significant contributions you'll be called on to make when you incorporate. Next, you'll have to decide how much you can cut your present take-home pay in order to divert money into the retirement plan. Your tax adviser and your bookkeeper can help you work up income figures, but only you and your wife can supply the key information: how much of that money you can do without.

There are often differences in the amounts the members of a group can put aside. In such a situation, some of the recommendations in Chapter 9 may help you.

2. *Mapping out the structure*. Part of the initial meeting is also devoted to the second step—the organization of the

corporation. Crawford asks his clients then to consider who will head the corporation, who will be on the board of directors, and who will be responsible for controlling patient flow, billing, and finances. Those decisions are crucial because the board of directors will make policy and the officers will carry it out. He also explains the various relationships of the doctors to the corporation and discusses the business reasons for making the change. While an unincorporated doctor is simply an entrepreneur from the business standpoint, an incorporated doctor is a shareholder, an employe, and a beneficiary of the retirement plan. He may also be a member of the board of directors, an officer of the corporation, and a trustee of the retirement plan.

Lamon covers that ground in his discussion of the documents he'll prepare. He believes that doctors should have two corporations—a professional one to handle the flow of money for practice income and expenses and a service corporation to own equipment and any real estate the doctors may have in connection with the practice. The professional corporation pays rent to the other corporation for the use of the equipment and the building.

3. Drawing up the legal documents. As soon as you give your lawyer the go-ahead to change your practice to a corporation, he'll start work on the papers. While you'll have little to do with the actual work, much of what's done depends on you. For instance, your lawyer must draw up a retirement program to meet your objectives.

The rules that will govern the corporation must be formalized in papers known as the certificate of incorporation and the bylaws. They, too, will depend on the decisions you make about the structure of your corporation. For example, the bylaws and articles of incorporation will spell out how much power the president of the corporation will have, how much will rest with the board of directors, and how much will remain with the other doctor-shareholders.

Lamon explains that, with some variations, every lawyer forming a professional corporation will also prepare papers to steer the corporation through the forthcoming organizational meetings and will draft employment contracts between the corporation and the doctors, sales and rental agreements for equipment already used in the practice, and buy-and-sell agreements to allow for disposal of stock when a doctor dies, retires, or wants to leave the group.

This third step could be the most time-consuming in the whole incorporation procedure. While the work itself could be done in a relatively short period, the time actually required will depend on how fast the lawyer can work and how many other things he has to do. So this step could take from a few weeks to a few months.

One thing that could hold up the drafting of the papers is the approval of the tax adviser. Some lawyers prefer to process the papers on their own, but Lamon and many others believe it's better to show the tax adviser drafts of all papers. Afterwards, Lamon holds a meeting with the adviser and goes over the papers. If the doctor can be there, so much the better, says Lamon, but getting three busy people together can cost still more time.

4. Filing the certificate of incorporation. This simple but important step is the legal formality announcing formation of your corporation—its birth certificate. Your lawyer will draft the certificate, usually a brief document, and send it to the state capital. In some cases, you may never even see the certificate before it's filed. Under New Jersey law, for instance, the lawyer can sign it. Pesin says he files the paper even before drafting the other documents. Lamon waits for approval of the papers from the tax adviser before filing the certificate.

5. Starting the corporate books. Unlike the filing of the certificate of incorporation, this step is no mere formality. It marks the physical separation of the corporation from the prior practice and will require additional work from your bookkeeper, your tax adviser, and maybe even from you. For a while, you may have to keep two sets of books, one for the corporation and another for the prior practice. You won't enter any new patients or suppliers in the old books, but you will have to keep tabs on collections and disbursements until those books are phased out. You must also start new account books for the corporation to show that all receipts and all accounts receivable for services rendered after incorporation belong to the corporation. Similarly, all bills from suppliers are to be paid by the corporation. One of the key requirements is that you start a new corporate checking account.

There are two ways of handling the accounts receivable for services rendered prior to incorporation. Many attorneys believe the corporation should simply take them over. Thus, the money becomes corporate income as it's collected and part of it can be put away in the retirement plan. In that case, any prior bills are paid by the corporation. An alternative is to deposit the collections in the old bank account. Bills incurred before formation of the corporation are paid out of those. What's left is income to the prior practice.

While sorting out the accounts is a chore, it shouldn't delay the setting up of your corporation. You can do your paper work while the attorney is preparing the legal documents.

6. *Notifying patients and suppliers.* Once your corporation has been formed, you must notify everyone with whom you have had business relationships. Crawford advocates a printed notice asking suppliers to bill the corporation. He says you should tell patients, too, but point out that it's just a business arrangement and that it will in no way change the physician-patient relationship.

7. *Holding organizational meetings.* Although the corporation comes into being when the certificate of incorporation is filed, and the bank account is opened, there remain the formalities of issuing stock certificates, approving the bylaws, electing the board of directors and officers, and signing the legal documents your lawyer has prepared.

While three meetings may technically be required to complete those formalities—one meeting each for the incorporators, the stockholders, and the board of directors—what usually happens is that there is one meeting broken up into several parts. Usually the lawyer has prepared the agenda and will be pushing papers in front of you to sign. If you've worked along with him at the earlier step when he prepared the documents, you probably won't even have to read them at the meeting. But make sure you know what you're signing. One of those papers will be an employment agreement setting forth how much pay you'll get. It may also regulate your vacation time and how much you'll be reimbursed for expenses.

The attorney will prepare minutes of the meetings for you to keep as part of the corporation's permanent records. You may have to show them to an Internal Revenue Service auditor someday if one ever wants to make sure

CHECKLIST FOR NEWLY INCORPORATED M.D.s

This summary of the steps that a corporation must take will help you make sure everything's been taken care of.

1. Open a corporate checking account, designating the employes authorized to sign checks.

2. Order new forms, letterheads, billheads, record sheets, etc., listing the corporate name.

3. Get a new employer identification number from the I.R.S.

4. Change telephone and other directory listings to corporate name.

5. Register in corporate name for unemployment and workmen's compensation; add doctor-employes, when required.

6. Apply for new Blue Shield number.

7. Notify carriers of office and malpractice insurance.

8. Set up business expense records for all employes who may have claims for reimbursement of auto mileage and other expenses.

9. Set up employe records for profit-sharing and other fringe benefit plans.

that you operate your practice as a true corporation.

With the formalities taken care of and the rest of the work that preceded it completed, a professional corporation is on its way. With the right legal, accounting, and retirement-planning help, it's almost a routine operation. Of course, that assumes there won't be any haggling over who is to run the corporation, how much each man is to get, and what goals the group is going to try for in its practice. Presumably, you will have ironed out most of those questions before you consider incorporation. If you haven't, incorporation may give you the opening you've needed to ease any problems that have been bothering you.

7 YOUR BUSINESS METHODS WILL HAVE TO MEASURE UP

Maybe you're already keeping minute records of employes' working time and maintaining an unbreachable wall between the money your practice owes you today and what you'll have coming from it next month. But if you aren't in fact running that precise an operation now, you'll have to change when you incorporate. So far as handling money is concerned, management men, lawyers, and accountants all give the incorporating physician advice that boils down to this: "Shape up."

That injunction has nothing to do with honesty in keeping tax records; by tax time, all but a small minority of M.D.s have their fiscal records in good order. What it means is that the professional corporation must keep meticulous, day-by-day records, because that's what all corporations must do. A professional corporation can't simply be a practice masquerading as a corporation;

it must be a corporation.

The way a corporation is set up has the greatest effect on whether it is indeed a corporation and can qualify for tax treatment as such. (For advice on setting up corporations, see previous chapter.) After the original organization, though, the way a corporation handles its business affairs has the next greatest influence on whether it can qualify as a true corporation. And it's in this second area where you, as a corporate employe and officer, will have the greatest responsibility. The organization of your corporation will presumably be handled by experts, but you must oversee its daily operation after the papers are filed.

How do you go about handling those daily details? "You set up machinery for the centralization of power," says Jack C. Pettee of Professional Management, Asheville, N.C. There's no need to think of this in Machiavellian terms. It simply means that the titles of your board chairman, president, secretary, and treasurer shouldn't be window dressing, but a reflection of actual and clearly defined duties.

The treasurer has nominal responsibility for most of the money-handling in a corporation, though he operates under guidelines set by the board of directors. As the man who's responsible for the corporate accounts, the treasurer should be the one who signs checks. If other officers and employes are empowered to sign checks too, the treasurer must ride herd on them. The other officers also have financial responsibilities in their own assigned areas. The president should have authority to carry out the board's policy directives in such areas as compensation. For example, if your group now horsetrades coverage and vacation schedules, you'll have to get used to submitting any conflicts to him for decision. Time off is, of course, an element of compensation.

Such formal division of duties shouldn't worry you unduly. If you've been able to resolve questions of time off, compensation, and check-signing amicably enough in the past, there's no reason why things shouldn't run just as smoothly after you incorporate. "Somebody's been minding the store all along," Pettee observes. The only difference: Informal arrangements must be made formal.

Incorporation does add some new housekeeping chores for the officers, points out management consultant Nelson J. Young of PM Florida—East Coast, Miami. For example, you'll have to:

Make regular payments for pension and profit-sharing funds. You should plan ahead for these payments, whether you make periodic deposits to gain the advantages of dollar averaging or accumulate cash in a separate savings account to try to make deposits in the trust fund when the market is down. Either way, Young says, "These funds have to be in the trust before the end of the year."

Deposit tax money promptly after it's withheld. Because the doctors as well as their assistants are employes of a corporation, a good deal of money is withheld from salaries for income and Social Security taxes. Under the regulations, the corporation might have to deposit the taxes as often as once a week, and the Internal Revenue Service has begun to levy penalties on taxpayers who fail to meet the deadlines.

File additional tax returns. Both the corporation and the retirement trust must file returns—even though the corporation may not owe any taxes, and the trust certainly won't. If your corporation decides on a self-administered trust, the job of filing the trust's returns will be yours.

It's worth noting that the business chores you do as a corporate officer may lighten your work when you come to filing your own tax return. For instance, you won't have to make quarterly tax payments on your practice income, if you adjust your withholding to cover all the tax you'll owe. And your own tax return will be simpler to file when your salary and withheld taxes are neatly summarized on the Form W-2 from your corporation.

But as Nelson Young says, "In a professional corporation, some damn fool complication is always coming up. You can't pin them all down."

Several management men underscore the fact that switching to a corporate form will compel use of the precise business methods that doctors should probably have been employing right along. Richard V. Bibbero of Medical Management Control, San Francisco, stresses what he calls "fiscal preplanning" because, he says, "I don't like to say 'budgeting.' But that's really what it amounts to. A corporation should plan all of its finances very carefully to reduce its profit at the end of the year." In common with many attorneys and consultants, Bibbero favors showing as little profit as possible on a corporation's books, because the corporation with a profit will have to pay taxes. If some of the corporate earnings are later passed on to the stockholders, they'll have to pay a second tax on those "dividends."

Year-end bonuses are a natural way to case the problem. But Nelson Young warns that relying too heavily on bonuses can prove to be a trap. "The reason," he says, "is that bonuses are subject to caprice or control of stockholder-employes. Too much tinkering with bonuses could raise questions about the validity of the corporate entity."

Spending corporate income is one of a twinned pair of

problems. The other, paradoxically, is making sure your corporation has sufficient cash flow. Young warns that the higher legal and accounting costs of corporate practice—he estimates that they'll be at least 25 per cent higher than were noncorporate costs—may put a strain on finances. One solution is to borrow money. Since the corporation is likely to have limited assets, banks will probably require at least one of the physician-officers to cosign the note. Most lawyers and management consultants agree that such cosignatures won't jeopardize the corporation's tax status as a true corporation.* "Businessmen make a practice of cosigning their corporations' notes all the time," Pettee says.

Another way to assure that the firm has adequate capital is for the doctor-incorporators to put it up themselves. That's not a happy solution to the problem, because by adding capital the stockholders would in effect be making a long-term loan to themselves at no interest. But if the corporation is often caught in a cash squeeze, an ante from the M.D.s may be preferable to repeated borrowing, especially in periods like the present when money is hard to get and costly.

Any capital a doctor puts into the corporation will, of course, affect the value of the shares. Most attorneys and management men agree that shares should be valued at "book"—the value of the corporation's physical assets and capital. The shares should be revalued at least annually, and a buy-and-sell agreement among the stockholders is essential.

**Among the dissenters: Harry V. Lamon, an Atlanta attorney. "In the Holder case," he says, "a point was made of the fact that no cosignatures were given." As attorney in that case, Lamon defeated an I.R.S. contention that Dr. James S. Holder was not a corporate employe for tax purposes.*

The fact that a doctor has put his basic practice into a corporation doesn't limit what he does in his noncorporate hours. Unless the corporate agreement is specifically drawn to bar it, he may conduct his own practice, completely separate from the corporate practice. Such a side practice may help resolve conflicts between doctors whose individual requirements differ. In fact, it's entirely possible for a moonlighting doctor to have both a corporate profit-sharing plan and his own Keogh plan covering his individual practice. Who says that corporate life has to be regimented?

8 WHAT YOU CAN TAX-SHELTER IN A CORPORATE RETIREMENT PLAN

Since the Pension Reform Act of 1974 became law, there's been a lot of hand wringing among professional people about the new limits on contributions to corporate retirement plans. But now that the experts have had a long second look, it's clear that most physicians will be able to work within the restrictions to build a retirement plan that's as good or even better than before.

If you're already incorporated, you and your corporation advisers will have to rewrite your retirement plan to make the technical changes required by the new law. So now is the time to make sure you're using the right options.

A little analysis will clear up any confusion (see the box on pages 82-83). When you're checking your options, keep in mind that there's nothing to stop you from switching your plan now or later on to fit your needs. Whatever changes you decide on, they're likely to be important enough for you to make sure that your lawyer gets the Internal Revenue Service to approve them. If you have a master or prototype corporation plan, such as one through a mutual fund or insurance company, the procedure may be simpler.

Whether you're incorporated now, or considering the move, you'll want to make your choice of options on the basis of where you stand in your career. (But remember that you may be in a special situation where you'll need to make some choices that are out of the usual mold.) Here are a doctor's options based on age—and the personal situation that usually goes with that stage of his career:

Doctors in their 30s: Keep it simple

If you're in this age-group, your best bet is what the new law calls a *defined-contribution plan,* in which your corporation puts away an amount based on a percentage of your salary. You can do this with (1) a money-purchase plan in which the percentage is fixed; (2) a profit-sharing plan that allows you to vary the percentage from year to year; or (3) a combination of both. This arrangement requires no complicated formulas to figure out the contributions for you and the rest of the staff.

Here's how the defined-contribution plan works: Let's say your annual corporate salary is $60,000 and you have a money-purchase plan that calls for a contribution of 10 per cent. The sum of $6,000 goes into your retirement plan for you annually. Then, if you also have a profit-sharing plan, the corporation can put away an additional amount up to 15 per cent, or $9,000. Except for a special wrinkle explained in the box on pages 82-83, the corporation contributes the same percentage for your corporation's other employes.

Since the new limits went into effect in 1976, the annual

ceiling on total tax-deductible contributions to money-purchase and profit-sharing plans is 25 per cent of salary up to a maximum of $26,825 per participant. (The dollar limit is scheduled to rise periodically to keep pace with inflation.) You can build up your retirement fund even more by making a voluntary contribution out of your aftertax income, but anything over 6 per cent of your annual salary will be subtracted from the corporation's $26,825 maximum contribution. Forfeitures—money left behind by employes who leave—will also be subtracted from the corporation's contributions to a profit-sharing plan if they push the annual additions over the maximum. The forfeitures are subtracted from the contributions to money-purchase plans even when you're not putting in the maximum allowed.

Should you worry about how you'll make out under the new corporate retirement limitations in the 30s age-group? Not for a minute—time is on your side. Barring a roaring inflation for many years or some other economic catastrophe, you should do just fine. Assuming you're in your mid-30s and you put away $10,000 a year—well below the maximum—from now until you retire, you'll end up with more than $1,000,000 at age 65. Even if you wait 10 years or so until your earnings increase and thereafter put away $25,000 a year until you retire, you'll still end up with more than $1,000,000. That's based on bank interest now paid on long-term deposits. If your retirement fund earns more, you'll have an even bigger nest egg. (For exact figures see the box on pages 90-91.)

Within the limits, you can tailor the defined-contribution approach to your specific needs. You can have a money-purchase plan alone and contribute any amount up to the 25 per cent and $26,825 limit. Remember, though, that you must fix the contribution in advance, so you'll have to put away the money in lean years as well as in fat ones. Against that disadvantage, you'll get the advantage of saving administrative costs by having only one plan.

You can opt for a profit-sharing plan alone and have complete flexibility over the amount you contribute, but

---

COST-CUTTING OPTIONS TO HELP YOUR FUND GROW FASTER

The new pension law retains the major ways of reducing the cost of contributions for your employes. (For details, see Chapter 12.) Although you may not want to push the savings to the limit, you'll want to check out your plan—especially if you have a large payroll—to make sure you aren't putting away more than you need to. Some tips:

Stretch out vesting. Vesting is another word for ownership. You're allowed to stretch out the vesting so that employes can take out only a small share of the money put in for them if they leave the corporation after a short time. The new law permits several different methods of vesting and even allows no vesting for four years. However, if you want to give your employes an idea that benefits won't be deferred beyond reach, you'll probably choose a plan that assures them an increasing share of the money in their accounts at the rate of 10 per cent a year. Thus, if an employe left after two years, he could take 20 per cent of his money; after three years, he could take 30 per cent, and so on. The money the employe leaves behind is forfeited.

This and other approaches to vesting schedules have always been permitted. In practice, however, local I.R.S. offices often required physicians to use the most generous schedules. It's not clear at this point whether you'll be able to switch from a fast schedule—5 years, for example—to a 10-year plan, but it's worth looking into. If you can arrange it, however, you'll have to immediately vest all the money that's been put away up to now.

there's a disadvantage in that the maximum annual contribution in a profit-sharing plan is limited to 15 per cent of your pay. In that case, you could make a voluntary contribution of up to 10 per cent of your pay.

With a combination of money-purchase and profit-sharing, you can have flexibility, plus the right to contribute

---

Integrate your plan with Social Security. A professional corporation can credit part of the money paid to the Government's retirement plan as contributions to its own plan. That's retirement plan integration. It's permitted in both defined-contribution plans and defined-benefit plans, but in different ways. In a defined-contribution plan, the money paid to Social Security is subtracted from the amount the corporation contributes to its own plan each year; this results in an advantage for the highly paid employes. In a defined-benefit plan, the eventual Social Security payments are subtracted from the projected corporate retirement payments. Either way, integration of the plans serves to reduce the amount you put away for lower-paid and younger employes, so you stand to gain.

Restrict participation. Chances are your corporate retirement plan provides for the exclusion of part-timers (defined under the new law as anyone who works less than 1,000 hours a year) or short-timers (generally those who've been with you less than a year). What you may not realize is that you can also omit some regular employes on the basis of their age or the job they're in. For example, a corporation with four or five employes (including the doctors) might be able to limit the number of participants in the plan to three. Larger corporations can restrict the number of plan participants by about the same proportion.

One caution: Eliminating employes on the basis of age or job classification is a tricky business. The corporation must maintain a minimum percentage of participants. So if you cut it too closely and the percentage of participation drops below the required number because one or two participating employes leave, your plan could be disqualified.

the tax-deductible maximum (25 per cent or $26,825). The money-purchase contribution can be set at, say, 10 or 15 per cent. Then each year you can decide how much more you want to put into the profit-sharing plan. You can skip it altogether or put in any amount up to the legal limit. For that flexibility, though, you'll have to pay the cost of running two plans. Since administration will be more complicated under the new law, that could be a significant factor. So go over the figures with your advisers and see what you'll have to pay for flexibility.

Doctors in midcareer: All options open

At this stage in your career, you may find that the 25 per cent and $26,825 limits aren't too restrictive. And if you're not burdened by the contributions for your employes, which have to be roughly the same percentage as for you, then you may be satisfied with a defined-contribution program.

However, there's another approach that may let you put away more money for yourself and probably save you money on contributions for your employes. This method is called a *defined-benefit plan*. The details of defined-benefit plans are complicated, but the following basic points will help you decide if the idea is worth investigating further.

You start out by choosing the amount of annual retirement income you want—the defined benefit. That amount can be anything up to 100 per cent of your current annual salary, but not more than $80,475 a year. (Like the limit on defined contribution plans, this can rise, too.) After you settle on the retirement benefit, an actuary computes how much you have to put away each year to accumulate the fund you'll need at retirement to pay the benefit you want. The closer you are to retirement, the more the corporation can—in fact, must—put in each year to accumulate the fund you need. Since the odds are that you'll be older than the office staff, the contribution for you should be proportionately higher than for them. However, some of the advantage will be used up in the extra administrative costs of such plans.

There are two ways of using the defined-benefit approach. One is called a target-benefit plan, and the other is a fixed-benefit plan. Each has its own advantages and drawbacks. In the target-benefit arrangement, any investment earnings of the retirement fund in excess of or below the actuary's projection will fatten or decrease your projected retirement benefit. Since the actuary usually assumes that earnings will be at a modest level, typically 5 to 6 per cent, you'll usually end up with more than your plan calls for. However, contributions to a target plan are subject to a yearly $26,825 or 25 per cent limit, just the same as defined-contribution plans.

In the second approach, the fixed-benefit plan, any earnings in excess of the projected amount reduce the contributions. If earnings fall short, though, the corporation will have to make up the difference, so that your retirement benefit comes out as projected if you continue to work and earn at the projected level. But a fixed-benefit plan has the big advantage of greater leeway on contributions. Each year the corporation contributes whatever is necessary to build up the fund needed to provide the retirement benefit.

Here, according to Paul Brady of Pension Administrators, Inc., Ridgewood, N.J., is how the target type of defined-benefit plan would work out if you're a physician of 45 and getting a corporate salary of $60,000 a year: Assuming you wanted to put away the maximum $15,000 a year, you'd build up a fund that would pay out a retirement benefit of

$46,200 a year—with $42,000 from your savings and the balance from Social Security. That also assumes the retirement fund earned 5½ per cent annually. If it earned 7½ per cent, say, you'd have 20 per cent more at retirement. (In the fixed type of defined-benefit plan, the higher earnings would reduce the annual contribution.) You could increase your benefit even more with voluntary contributions.

The contribution for you, in this example, is at the rate of 25 per cent of your salary. However, for a 30-year-old nurse earning $7,500 a year, the contribution would come to only $497, or less than 7 per cent of her salary. For a 35-year-old

MERGE KEOGH INTO A CORPORATE RETIREMENT PLAN?

What's the best thing to do with your Keogh plan if you switch from self-employed to corporate status and set up a new retirement plan under the more liberal rules governing professional corporations? Many believe that you had little choice but to freeze your Keogh plan money—that is, keep the plan intact but make no further contributions to it. It turns out, though, that you do have a choice. It even sounds attractive enough on the surface to lure some doctors in. But beware: It's so fenced in with restrictions that you'll probably be better off to pass it up.

The new choice stems from a private ruling by Isidore Goodman, head of the I.R.S. pension and trust branch, indicating that Keogh plan assets can be transferred to a corporate retirement plan.

That sounded like good news for doctors who wanted to avoid duplicating trustee fees for *two* retirement plan funds after incorporating. It sounded like good news, too, for those who prefer to act as their own trustees. (For Keogh plans there must earning $7,500, the contribution would be $674, or less than 9 per cent.

Savings on contributions for your staff may well make this approach attractive. The greater the spread between your age and the ages of the staff, the more these savings are likely to be. If everyone stayed to retirement, the contribution levels would even out, and everyone would get the same percentage of retirement pay. But since most staff members leave well before that time, your savings are a permanent gain.

A final word on this type of defined-benefit plan: Even

---

be a corporate trustee such as a bank or insurance company, while an owner of a professional corporation may act as his own trustee.)

Later clarification by Goodman of some points that were left vague in his ruling, however, threw cold water on the hopes that had been raised. It turns out that Keogh assets can be transferred to a corporate plan only if the corporate plan has a bank trustee. Once transferred, the Keogh assets must be kept separate from the corporate plan assets and are still subject to all the restrictions of Keogh plans—e.g., no distributions before age 59½.

Even for those who already have a bank trustee or are willing to change their corporate plan so that it would have a bank trustee, there are hitches that argue against a transfer. Costly paper work is involved—filings with the I.R.S. and, possibly, amending the corporate plan.

There's hope that eventually the I.R.S. may issue rules that make it a simple matter to merge Keogh assets into a corporate plan. Until then, the difficulties of a transfer may outweigh whatever small savings in administrative charges might be realized.

though the plan is based on the amount needed to fund an annual retirement benefit, you're not restricted to that form of payout. You can decide to take your money in a lump sum or in a few large installments. You don't have to make your decision until retirement, when you'll have a better idea of your needs and your tax situation.

Doctors in their 50s and 60s: Make up for lost time

If you're in this age bracket, the new law provides you with a perfect opportunity to catch up on your retirement saving by using two plans at once. You can adopt a fixed-benefit pension plan and put away whatever's needed to fund an annual retirement benefit of up to 100 per cent of your salary to a maximum of $80,475 a year. On top of that, you can put away an additional 10 per cent of your salary in a defined-contribution plan.

According to Paul Brady, if you're 55 you can tax-shelter almost as much as you're paid each year. For example, if you could live on a salary of $40,000 a year, your corporation can put away $30,165 for you in a fixed-benefit plan and $4,000 more in a money-purchase plan. In just 10 years, you'd have more than half a million dollars in your retirement plans. While putting away all that money for you, the corporation will have to contribute only $1,246 for a 30-year-old nurse earning $7,500 a year and $1,470 for a 35-year-old nurse.

To sum up: Whatever your age or your situation, it's clear that there are still generous allowances for everyone even under the restrictions of the new law. You'll have to work out the details with your own advisers, of course. Remember that earnings on the money contributed to a retirement plan aren't taxed until the benefits are paid. And if you die before you retire, your family can collect the money from a corporate retirement plan free of Federal estate tax, provided it's paid directly to them or into a trust. The new law hasn't changed any of that.

HOW RETIREMENT PLANS COMPARE

		What the corporation can contribute
DEFINED-CONTRIBUTION PLANS	Money-purchase	Up to 25% of compensation (fixed in advance), maximum of $26,825*
	Profit-sharing	Up to 15% of compensation (variable each year), maximum of $26,825*
	Combined money-purchase and profit-sharing	Up to 25% of compensation (partially fixed and partially variable), maximum of $26,825*
DEFINED-BENEFIT PLANS	Fixed-benefit	Amount needed to fund predetermined benefit, no maximum
	Target-benefit	Amount needed to fund predetermined benefit, up to maximum of 25% of compensation or $26,825 per year*
DOUBLE PLAN	Money-purchase	Up to 10% of compensation (fixed in advance)
	and fixed-benefit	Amount needed to fund predetermined benefit, no maximum

**To be increased to keep pace with inflation.*

UNDER THE NEW LAW

	What happens to forfeitures when employes leave	What happens to annual investment earnings or losses	What you get at retirement
	Corporate contributions reduced	Added to or subtracted from account balances	Balance of account
	Added to remaining account balances	Added to or subtracted from account balances	Balance of account
	Corporate contributions reduced if they are at maximum; otherwise, added to profit-sharing accounts	Added to or subtracted from account balances	Balance of account
	Corporate contributions reduced	Annual corporate contributions adjusted to reflect them	Predetermined amount, up to 100% of compensation, maximum of $80,475 per year*
	Corporate contributions reduced	Added to or subtracted from account balances	Predetermined amount, up to 100% of compensation, maximum of $80,475 per year* plus or minus investment gains and losses
	Corporate contributions reduced	Added to or subtracted from account balances	Balance of account
	Corporate contributions reduced	Annual corporate contributions adjusted to reflect them	Predetermined amount, up to 100% of compensation, maximum of $80,475 per year*

9 EXTRA FLEXIBILITY FOR YOUR CORPORATE RETIREMENT PLAN

"I'm so strapped for cash these days," one incorporated-group doctor announces, "I'd like to cut down the amount of money we put away in the retirement fund this year."

"Cut down!" another man in the same group retorts, "I wish there were some way to *increase* the contributions!"

And so it goes as doctors find themselves trapped in the lockstep of a corporate retirement savings program that requires the same contribution for each. A similar conflict can occur with partners who are considering incorporation of their practice.

Take the most common instance of the problem: A corporation has a money-purchase and a profit-sharing plan allowing a total contribution of 25 per cent of salary. There are two doctors in the corporation, and each has $60,000 a year of earnings to divide between salary and a retirement plan contribution. Each doctor can draw $48,000 pay and have $12,000 put away in the retirement plans. The trouble arises when one man wants to have more pay and the other wants the maximum put away toward retirement.

Some solutions to the problem are still in the gray area of the developing law on professional corporations. Other solutions are simply too expensive, and some aren't practical for most doctors. Still, drastic problems often call for drastic remedies, so if you and your corporate colleagues can't agree on how much to put away under the usual pension arrangements, consider the following four possible solutions.

Option out of the plan. This is one of the simplest and most widespread ways of giving one man more current income. The doctor simply elects not to participate in all or part of the corporate retirement program. One of the ways he can option out is by signing a form stating that he doesn't want the corporation to make contributions for him in, say, the profit-sharing plan. The Internal Revenue Service doesn't object if a doctor wants to do that.

The I.R.S. could object, though, if that money were paid out as current income in lieu of the corporate contribution—without a good business reason. That's because the payment would give the doctor a choice the office staff doesn't have; in effect, it would discriminate against those employes. And if you have a very small corporation, this solution might result in participation dropping below the allowable level.

Since the point of optioning out of the retirement plan is to give the money to the doctor currently, the problem is how to do it with a valid reason. One way would be to set the salary on the basis of productivity—assuming the doctor who wants more is in fact a bigger producer. Caution: You may be forced to prove you acted for a good business reason if the I.R.S. questions the arrangement.

Omit contributions on bonuses. This solution can shift a limited amount of cash into the current pay of a doctor who needs it. Here's how that works: The retirement plan will specify that contributions are to be computed on basic salary only—with bonuses excluded. If each man has $60,000 a year of earnings to divide between salary and retirement plan contributions, the doctor who wants to put away the maximum might take a salary of $48,000, and the corporation would put away $12,000 in a money-purchase and profit-sharing plan. A doctor who wants to put away less might get a salary of $30,000, a retirement plan contribution of $7,500, and a bonus of $22,500.

Although both doctors have a total of $60,000 a year, the one with the bonus gets $4,500 more pay than the other and, of course, has $4,500 less put away in the retirement plan. Although that arrangement is considered legal, many lawyers advise you not to push it too far. How far is too far? Perhaps only the I.R.S. knows, but setting one salary about 50 to 60 per cent higher than the other, as in the example above, seems fairly safe. You also have to make sure you don't discriminate against the office staff; you can't reduce the contribution you make for them.

Form separate corporations. That's probably the safest way to achieve the desired mix of current pay and retirement contributions. What happens is that the physicians in an incorporated group terminate their current relationship, with each of them forming a corporation. Then the corporations form a joint venture to continue the practice.

The major drawback to this arrangement is cost. Each corporation would have to pay separate annual legal and accounting fees, in addition to the large outlays needed to start separate corporations and establish separate retirement plans.

Many group doctors have tried a cheaper variation on that "separate corporation" setup, but it involves the risk of a double tax bill if the I.R.S. challenges it. The idea is to have the doctor who's interested in making hefty contributions to his group retirement program incorporate while the others remain unincorporated and stick with Keogh plans. The problem with this arrangement is that the doctor who's incorporated hasn't really changed his basic relationship with the former partnership. In a future audit, the I.R.S. could choose to call his corporation a sham and kill his retirement plan—with an immediate tax bill on the contributions and earnings.

Allow early withdrawal of retirement funds. This way of easing the need for cash involves letting employes borrow money or permitting payouts for emergencies such as the purchase of a house or other large expenditures. However, if you start borrowing and paying back money to a retirement plan as if you were dealing with your local loan company, the I.R.S. could blow the whistle on the grounds that you're thwarting the purpose of the plan. Many I.R.S. districts require a plan to specify that you must repay a loan from it within three years, that you can't reborrow it once it's paid back, and that you provide adequate security. And remember that what you do for the corporation doctors you have to do for the employes. For example, if you permit payment of money for doctors' emergencies, you'll have to do the same for all.

As you can see, if you and your corporate colleagues can't agree on a uniform level of retirement plan contributions, it's worth exploring the solutions. And don't forget that there's one foolproof solution often overlooked: the defined-benefit pension plan approach. Such plans *require* larger contributions for an older man—usually the one who wants to put away the heftier contributions anyway. (see Chapter 8.) So if the conflict over retirement plan contributions is a matter of age, you may have a ready-made answer.

Should you consider using a ready-made retirement plan?

To do its tax-deferring job well, a retirement plan must fit the requirements of the particular corporation that sets it up. But that doesn't mean you have no alternative to having a plan drawn up specifically for your corporation. There are, in fact, hundreds of alternatives.

They're the master plans banks, insurance companies, mutual funds, and other organizations have designed. Collectively, these prepackaged plans offer a wide variety of investment media and funding methods, and the basic format of each plan has already been approved by the Internal Revenue Service.

Some master plans offer several fundamentally different options; others permit only minor variations. You and your lawyer need only select the options or variations that fit your corporation. The basic retirement plan is ready-drafted. You and your advisers check the options and mark off the choices that suit your situation.

A lot depends on beginning with the right plan, but there are many to choose from. For example, at one stroke some years ago, the Internal Revenue Service qualified 734 master plans for tax-deductible treatment. New ones have been coming along almost daily since, and master plans already in existence are being amplified to give you more choices. At last count, there were thousands of different sponsors of master plans, several offering more than one kind of plan.

Whether you choose a master plan or an individually tailored one, your attorney or the retirement specialist he brings in will do the same groundwork to get you through the basic incorporation steps. Up to then, your attorney's fee will be substantially the same regardless of what you decide to do. But if your next step is to choose a master plan instead of a custom-designed one, a quick survey of attorneys in New York, Georgia, Texas, Illinois, and California indicates that you can save a substantial amount of legal fees.

Another advantage of a master plan is that it's already qualified for tax-deductible treatment by the I.R.S. An individually tailored plan, as an entirely new document, must be reviewed in detail. But the sponsors of a master plan merely submit what's called a "joinder," spelling out the options you've picked. That's what the I.R.S. usually concentrates on, not the main body of the plan that it has already qualified. So it's not only easier to go the master plan route, it'll probably take less time. One big disadvantage of most such plans is that your investments are usually tied to the sponsor's product—mutual fund, insurance, or whatever.

There may be another saving if you and your attorney decide to use a master plan offered by a retirement-plan servicing organization that provides actuarial analysis. Such an organization can do a feasibility study and compute the contributions you'll have to make to meet your retirement objectives. Buying those services in a package with the plan may cost less than you'd have to pay separately to an attorney and an actuary. Here, for example, is the fee structure of Certified Plans, a California-based retirement planning and administrative firm. There's a basic setup charge of $500, plus $25 per participant for each of the first 25. The charge per person is scaled down if more than 25 enter the plan. Thus, charges for a typical four-man corporation with an office staff of six would run $750. (It would be more if there were two plans.) "We work with the client, his accountant, and his attorney," explains Charles R. Billman of Certified Plans. "We review the data sheet that lists employes' ages, incomes, and years of service, plus various options they want. Then the actuaries work up that information and we develop a complete retirement-plan package for their consideration, fitting it into one of our master plans."

If you're seriously considering using a master plan, you or your attorney will want to look at what's available. You might check the trust department of your local bank and ask if it has a master corporate retirement plan. Just as close to home, your life insurance agent or even your securities dealer may offer a master plan. Once you've got several plans in hand, you'll want some means of telling them apart and judging which is best for you.

Here are the questions that can help you decide whether a particular master plan is right for your needs or not.

How much choice does it give you among types of retirement plans? Some master plans offer a limited choice and some don't even offer any. You may have to take a profit-sharing plan or nothing. Others don't offer a defined benefit plan.

The plans vary greatly in detail—and some of those variations may be important to you. For example, some master plans don't permit integration with Social Security.*

How responsive is a master plan to your needs? There are two basic types of master plans to choose from. The variable plan offers many options and is highly flexible; the standard plan is inflexible and spells out precisely what you can and can't do in your retirement plan.

For instance, a master plan may require immediate and full vesting of all employes' benefits. That means that the employe can take out whatever the corporation has contributed to the retirement plan for him when he leaves. Thus, there's no motivation for him to stay with the corporation on a long-term basis. Such a plan also eliminates all forfeitures, or "fall-ins," from employes—usually nonprofessionals who work for the corporation a few years and then leave. That money might otherwise be allocated to the accounts of the long-term employes—the M.D.s, presumably, and the career assistants who remain with the corporation. Or it can reduce future corporate deposits.

A standard plan also may not permit the restrictions you'd like to put on which employes are to be covered by the plan. Further, it might also force you to set an immutable formula for contributions to a profit-sharing plan. If so, you can't change the contribution percentage from year to year, regardless of what happens to your corporation's income and expenses.

**In an integrated plan, the corporation counts part of the Social Security payments either toward its contribution or toward the pension benefits and, thus, lowers the cost of covering the office staff.*

Another potential problem with a standard plan may crop up if the plan gives a bank the investment authority for a retirement fund's assets. For as Billman warns: "If you're not a big corporation, the bank may want to put you into its common trust fund, and the performance of those funds has been mixed."

Who will invest your retirement funds? A refinement of the master plan, called a "prototype," may offer a solution if you prefer not to have a bank determining your investments. The difference between a prototype and a master plan, in practice, is that in a master plan, the sponsoring financial institution names the trustee—usually a trust company or a bank. In a prototype plan, the professional corporation selects its own trustee—not necessarily a bank. The trustee may instead be one or more individuals, who can be officers of the corporation. Thus, you can name yourself as trustee, and then make all the investment decisions for your retirement fund—subject, of course, to the limitations imposed by the plan itself.

Obviously, you'll save the trustee's fee if you're in charge. But there may be advantages in flexibility, too. Energy Fund's prototype plan, for example, permits the trustee to use insurance and annuities as the investment medium for up to 49 per cent of the annual contribution—the maximum under I.R.S. regulations. The Dreyfus prototype limits the amount you can put into ordinary life insurance to a maximum of 25 per cent of the annual contribution.

How will your retirement funds be invested? Mutual funds, banks, and insurance companies ordinarily don't charge for their master plans, and this fact will influence how your retirement plan invests its funds. Obviously, these financial institutions will have to get their revenues other ways. This they do either from commissions on the sale of equities or insurance to your retirement fund, or from investment management fees (on a bank's common trust fund, for example).

"When you go into a master plan," says Jack McKinley, president of the New York-based McKinley & Co., which surveys such plans and matches them to the retirement needs of corporations, "your retirement funds are likely to be tied to the assets its sponsor sells; those assets may be units in a bank's common trust fund, shares of a mutual fund, or annuities or life insurance from an insurance company." Most funds with plans therefore require you to invest in their fund shares except for the amounts their plans permit you to put into some form of insurance. And insurance company master plans provide that part of your annual contribution must go into some kind of insurance contract. Sometimes they provide for investment of the balance in the shares of an associated mutual fund and sometimes, as with The Guardian Life Insurance Company of America and Safeco Securities, Inc., you get wide investment latitude.

For even more investment freedom, however, you may want to go to a master plan offered by an independent organization. A securities dealer like Merrill Lynch, Pierce, Fenner & Smith Inc. lets you invest in a wide range of different kinds of assets, from stocks and bonds to real estate. A retirement planning and administrative service like Certified Plans, Inc., sells no assets at all. Or you may find a rare master plan like the one offered by Marine Midland Bank of New York, which contains a wide-open investment option letting you put your retirement funds into any kind of asset you choose.

Being locked into a sponsor's specific investment medium can create problems, warns Atlanta attorney Harry V. Lamon Jr. One danger: Your retirement income might be fixed for life by the level of the stock market on the date when you retire. You'd be in trouble if that date coincided with a bear market such as some we've been forced to go through. And Billman adds a warning: "If you'd used a master plan that required you to put your money in a mutual fund, you could lose a substantial portion of your assets in a bear market." If you wanted to change funding mediums because of poor performance, you'd have to change master plans. And that's a very difficult thing to do, say both men. Recognizing the problem, The Side Fund lets you buy shares of other mutual funds after two years in its master plan, provided at least 50 per cent of plan assets are invested in The Side Fund at all times.

In sum, there's a wide choice among master plans, and some offer a high degree of adaptability. But it's difficult to find a master plan that offers complete investment freedom combined with precise tailoring to the requirements of your corporation and its employes. For that combination, your best bet is a plan drafted specially for your own corporation.

11 RUNNING CORPORATE PENSION PLANS: WHAT HELP IS NEEDED?

Despite repeated entreaties, a two-man Eastern corporation formed three years ago still has most of its pension and profit-sharing money parked in savings accounts. At first the two physicians were simply undecided about what to do. Now, with deposits approaching $100,000, they're too awed by the size of their bankroll to "play with the money," as they put it.

What they've done is to cop out on the important job of investing their retirement funds. As a result, they're cheating themselves and their employes out of money they'd have if they were getting a better return. An isolated case? Unfortunately not. All too many doctors I've come across are either too busy, too uninformed, or too careless to manage their retirement plans properly.

What's more, investments aren't the only part of the job that many doctors let slide: There's a whole series of interrelated tasks that have been multiplied and complicated by the Pension Reform Act of 1974. Someone has to keep records of contributions, income, and gains, and the money has to be allocated among participating corporate employes. Complicated reports must be filed with the Internal Revenue Service and the Department of Labor. And finally, employes should be informed of their account balances, and the programs should be explained in a way that makes the benefits meaningful to them.

If you're in corporate practice, you've got to see that these jobs are done. You may decide to get help for every last detail, or you may decide that you'll shoulder much of the load. Whatever you choose to do, remember that the way your plan is managed will determine how successful it is in insuring a financially secure retirement and how bothered you'll be with legal and personnel problems. Three management styles that will help crystallize your own approach to this problem are explained below.

Luxury-class management

You don't have to get involved in the operations of your corporation's pension and profit-sharing plans, provided you're willing to pay for being a gentleman trustee. You can retain an investment counselor or get a bank trust department to handle investments. You can get a pension actuary to keep the records, allocate the money, and file the reports. And, finally, you can delegate the responsibility of keeping your employes informed to a management consultant.

Going this route may be as much a matter of temperament as anything else. An ophthalmologist I know, who earns about $100,000 a year, has always relied heavily on professional help. He felt that there was even more reason to do so after he incorporated. "I'm an expert in medicine and leave business to the experts in that field," he told me.

The size of your practice is an important determinant of the approach you take. One doctor I've worked with loved to fool around with figures and to keep his finger on all the financial aspects of his practice. But when he incorporated and took in an associate, and the office staff grew to 10, it became apparent that keeping tabs on the retirement plans would be a full-time job. So he now contents himself with riding herd on the managers he's hired.

Just how much it will cost for a complete management package depends on factors such as the amount of money you've deposited in the accounts, the number of employes in your corporation, and the type of plan or plans you have.

Take the cost of investment management. Banks usually charge an annual fee of $5 per $1,000 of assets, so a corporation with $100,000 in its funds would pay $500 annually. The fee may be scaled down on large trusts, but there may be additional costs. Here are a couple of examples. The Wachovia Bank & Trust Company of Winston-Salem, N.C., has a minimum charge of $500 for one plan and $250 for each additional plan. The American Fletcher National Bank & Trust Company in Indianapolis has a different arrangement—$250 annual minimum fee per plan for individual management and $100 per plan if the money is invested in the bank's common trust fund—that's a pool of funds similar to a mutual fund.

In addition to investment services, banks generally also do some record-keeping for doctors and may even supply enough information to simplify tax-filing chores.

Investment counselors, on the other hand, usually confine their activities to their special field, some charging even more than the banks. For example, Lionel D. Edie & Company of New York City has a minimum fee of $250 a year and charges $1,000 to manage a $100,000 retirement fund. Stein Roe & Farnham of Chicago charges only $500 per $100,000, but has a minimum fee of $2,500 a year.

If you want somebody to do all the computations required to run a retirement plan, consider hiring a pension actuary. A typical firm is Consulting Actuaries, Inc., of Clifton, N.J. For $790 a year for a one-doctor corporation with three employes, the firm will administer a retirement program for a corporation that has a pension and a profit-sharing plan. For that money, the actuaries will figure out how much the corporation has to contribute for each employe under a defined or fixed-benefit plan. (Since that figure depends on the employe's age and pension goal, it requires an actuary's specialized skills.) If the corporation has a plan based on a percentage contribution, such as a profit-sharing or money-purchase pension plan, then the firm will allocate the contributions.

In addition, Consulting Actuaries figures out how to allocate earnings, gains, and forfeitures. A report is provided for the corporation as well as for each employe, and all tax forms are prepared. The actuary also handles the preparation of I.R.S. reports; with two plans, 10 have to be completed every year.

For all these services, the actuary's fee is a bargain—especially if your accountant is unable or unwilling to do the work. Remember, though, that the fee will depend on the number of doctors or employes in the corporation, as well as the number of plans.

Actuarial Systems, Inc., of San Jose, Calif., has a fee system that works a little differently. The minimum is $600

SOME PACKAGED PENSION PLANS HAVE BUILT-IN BUGS

You can probably get the investment, actuarial, and other services you need for a pension and profit-sharing plan cheaper if you buy them as a unit through a master or prototype plan. (For details, see Chapter 10.) Such plans are usually offered by insurance companies, banks, and mutual funds.

These services are offered cheaply because their sponsors are anxious to handle the investment of your money. In fact, many master and prototype plans lock you into a specific mutual fund or insurance plan. That's the most serious drawback to these arrangements. Once you put your money in, there's usually no way to change the investment program without starting all over with a new plan. Even if there are options, they may be too limited to meet changing conditions—a new colleague, for example, who wants to make his own investment choices.

Also, most such plans cannot be tailored to fit your needs, as can one that's individually drawn. A few concerns do offer wider choices. PRO Services of Flourtown, Pa., offers a package deal. Certified Plans, Inc., of Newport Beach, Calif., for example, gives a complete system package with its master pension and profit-sharing plans. To give investment flexibility, the company allows each participant to direct where its money is placed. This means you're not tied to a specific investment program but can move money from stocks, to bonds, to savings accounts at your heart's content. There's one catch, though. The package that Certified Plans offers is almost as expensive as the luxury-class management approaches you can put together yourself.

for two percentage contribution plans and $900 for a defined benefit and profit-sharing plan, plus one-tenth of 1 per cent of payroll. While this is a higher minimum than charged by many other consultants, the firm throws in extra consulting services.

The last major job that needs doing in any corporate practice is explaining benefits to employes. While you can't expect your office staff to accept retirement-plan contributions in lieu of current pay—they may never see the money, and they know it—you may get extra mileage in the form of loyalty and more willing work. The only way to do that is to explain to new employes what the program will do for them and to keep older employes informed of the progress of their accounts. And employes who are leaving must get a statement of their accounts that shows them how they stand on taxes.

For the personal touch on this job, you may need the services of a management consultant. He can put the pension and profit-sharing benefits in perspective so that employes understand what's being done for them and why. Typically, management consultants charge between $30 and $40 an hour for extra tasks that can add many hours to their annual services.

There's another system for getting outside management help for retirement funds; it involves choosing a master or prototype plan. These may offer fee savings, but with such serious drawbacks that many retirement-plan specialists don't recommend them. For details on this alternative, see the box on page 111 and the previous chapter.

Economy-class management

Many doctors may not need or want luxury-class help with

their retirement plans. "I tried it with a team of consultants," one doctor complained to me, "but they just got in each other's way." There are ways, however, to modify luxury arrangements to suit your own particular situation.

For example, a New York internist I work with has a stock broker who's tuned to his exact needs. The broker has been picking bonds yielding an average of 7½ per cent ever since the doctor incorporated three years ago, and he's satisfied with the growth of his retirement fund. "Some of my friends have been paying good money to investment counselors whose stock recommendations have gone sour," the doctor reported. He has an actuary to do all the paperwork.

Another doctor solved his management problem in a piecemeal fashion. He's got a top-notch accountant who's adapted his regular services to the needs of professional corporations; a special department does the actuarial work on pension and profit-sharing plans. In this way, the doctor gets his retirement-fund work done along with the general corporation work. Sure, he's paying for the additional accounting work, but he figures it's a lot less than he'd have to pay a separate consultant. To invest his money in stocks, he's found a bank with a top-notch common trust fund. That service costs him more than $1,000 a year, but he's counting on a 10 per cent growth rate and isn't worried.

Still another option for getting management of your retirement plan can tie in your insurance needs. Many insurance men are set up to handle actuarial services, and they'll do it at a bargain rate for customers because they can make money on the commissions. Vaughan-Kearney, Inc., of Ridgewood, N.J., does this job for a flat fee of $400 for two plans in the first year of operation and $500 a year thereafter.

Fly-it-yourself management

If you're interested in cutting down expenses, and your corporation is small enough—say two or three employes—you can drastically reduce the number of outsiders you need to hire. The only catch: You've got to be willing to pitch in. If you *prefer* to get involved, you may opt for this method just for the fun of it. That's the reason given by a doctor-friend of mine who says, "I enjoy watching the dividends and interest roll in, and I like making investment decisions." He keeps his records in apple-pie order, too.

No matter how good your records and how much work you're willing to do, you'll still need the help of an accountant or tax adviser with the forms required by the Internal Revenue Service. If only a few employes are involved, though, and you supply the records, you might be able to convince your accountant to do the work as an add-on to the rest of the job.

Whatever management style you decide to use, you should count on having an annual review by your regular tax advisers. If you're directly involved in the management of your fund, that's essential.

But even professional help is no guarantee of success. While reviewing the performance figures supplied by a bank to a medical corporation in Poughkeepsie, N.Y., I discovered that the pension fund had gotten a return of less than 2 per cent, and that the money-handling procedures were very shoddy. The corporation's doctor-president is now picking low-risk bonds with the help of a broker. He's earning over 7 per cent and paying no management fee at all.

12 How to Get the Most for Your Money

A major inducement for doctors to incorporate their practices is, of course, the advantageous retirement plans that incorporation makes possible. But to qualify for favorable tax treatment, retirement plans must cover the doctors' aides as well as the doctors. This means that they can be expensive, almost prohibitively so with a large staff.

The doctors, then, must try to hold costs in check. And there's a danger in that: They might—even inadvertently—become guilty in the eyes of the Internal Revenue Service of giving themselves retirement advantages they do not give their aides. That would be discriminatory and violate I.R.S. rules.

But there are ways, says Sanford L. Brickner, a Santa Ana, Calif., attorney, to remain generous to your aides, abide by I.R.S. rules, and still cut costs.

Brickner's knowledge of the ins and outs of professional

corporations is formidable. His own law firm, Block and Brickner, Inc., was the first professional corporation to be licensed in California. A certified public accountant as well as an attorney, he has formed hundreds of professional corporations and has designed retirement plans for medical corporations employing as few as one and as many as 80 doctors. In the following question-and-answer exchange with a Medical Economics editor, Brickner tells just how far a doctor can go toward reducing the cost of a retirement plan. He deals in outer limits, he says, but does so with this warning: Don't crowd those outer limits! Reaching too far, if it doesn't actually disqualify the retirement plan, can cost more in employe morale than it gains in financial benefits.

Q. *Mr. Brickner, are there any hard and fast rules by which an incorporating doctor can minimize the cost of his retirement plan?*

A. No. A number of factors combine to determine just what he'll get for his money. Doctors who are incorporating should learn what those factors are in order to assure themselves retirement plans that best suit their circumstances.

Q. *Isn't a major cost factor the number of people who will be covered by the plan?*

A. That's right. And tax laws say that a corporation's retirement plan must not discriminate in favor of stockholders, officers, or highly compensated employes; it must include all employes who qualify for it, regardless of the cost to the corporation.

Q. *Then would it be in an incorporating doctor's interest to limit the number of employes who qualify?*

A. Theoretically, yes. Practically, however, it may not be.

A retirement plan is a tremendously valuable and popular fringe benefit. By setting up one that goes out of its way to leave certain employes uncovered, a doctor might create a real morale problem; he might find it difficult in the future to attract the caliber of aide he needs, too.

Q. *Mightn't he also be guilty of discriminating?*

A. He might. But a retirement plan covering a number of employes could be prohibitively expensive. He can't just cover all employes automatically. He has to set up conditions for coverage that weed out some; at the same time, the plan must be fair—even generous—to his aides.

Q. *Isn't it asking a bit much for a plan to do all that?*

A. Well, yes. But it can be done, and within the law. Let me explain how in terms of outer limits—the limits to which a doctor can go to reduce his plan's cost without being guilty of discriminating.

Q. *Are you suggesting that he shoot for those outer limits?*

A. Not at all. I'm suggesting that he'd do well to learn the outer limits so that he won't run the risk of crossing them. The I.R.S. may disqualify his plan altogether if he pushes too far.

Q. *All right, where do we start?*

A. With a doctor who's just incorporated his practice and decided to establish a retirement trust, using a combined profit-sharing and pension plan. Let's say he's netting $50,000 before taxes and decides he can live on a $40,000 salary. That leaves him $10,000 a year to put into a retirement trust.

Q. *The question then is how much of that $10,000 is going to be for the doctor's benefit and how much must be allocated for the benefit of his employes?*

A. Exactly. And the decision must be made with the

no-discrimination rule in mind. The plan must be tested for discrimination in two basic areas—coverage and allocation of benefits among those covered.

Q. *You're saying that the plan does not have to cover all the corporation's employes?*

A. That's right. The I.R.S. provides several ways that employes may legitimately be excluded from coverage. There's the part-time exclusion, for example; say, for employes who work less than 1,000 hours a year.

Q. *Obviously, then, it would be to the doctor's advantage to have two aides, each working only 17½ hours a week, rather than one aide working 35 hours?*

A. For purposes of exclusion, yes, but a more important consideration is office efficiency. The Internal Revenue Code also lets us exclude employes who haven't been with the corporation a prescribed length of time—say one year.

Q. *But any waiting-period requirement would apply to the doctor as well as to his aides, wouldn't it?*

A. No. The plan could provide immediate coverage for all employes currently in the corporation, but make new ones wait.

Q. *Does age enter into it in any way?*

A. Yes. You can require that employes must be at least 25 to participate. Anyone younger wouldn't be eligible.

Q. *I see what you mean about outer limits. Are there other ways of holding down the number of employes covered?*

A. Oh, yes. For instance, the Revenue Code provides that a plan is not discriminatory if it covers 70 per cent of all employes. That's 70 per cent of all employes left after we've excluded part-timers and those who haven't satisfied the minimum age or waiting period.

Q. *Can you explain that with an example?*

A. All right, let's suppose we have a corporation employing 15—five doctors and 10 ancillary employes. Let's say that of those 15 we can exclude five either because they're part-timers or because they have not completed a full year's service on the last day of the year. That leaves 10. If our plan covers 70 per cent, or seven of them, we've met the statutory test of coverage.

Q. *But how might you legitimately exclude those other three employes?*

A. By wording the plan to exclude certain job classifications, such as receptionist. Let's say, anyway, that of 15 employes we now have only seven eligible for coverage.

Q. *And five of those seven are doctors?*

A. Five are doctors. Now the Revenue Code—and let me cite Section 401 of the Code for everything I've said thus far—states further that if we've made 70 per cent of all employes *eligible* for coverage, we must cover at least 80 per cent of those eligible.

Q. *You're saying that we don't have to cover even seven?*

A. That's right. Once we've made 70 per cent eligible, you see, we can introduce other preconditions to their membership in the plan. A common one is requiring that an employe contribute a percentage of his salary before he shares in what the corporation contributes. That employe contribution percentage might go as high as 6 per cent.

Q. *The 80 per cent of 70 per cent rule means that we have to cover at least six persons in your example–80 per cent of 7 equals 5.6. So can we assume that one employe disqualifies himself for coverage by refusing to contribute the called-for percentage?*

A. All right. That would leave us covering only six of our 15 employes. But we need to be careful here. The regulations say that requiring participating employes to kick in as much as 6 per cent of their salaries may not be bad. However, a requirement of even 2 per cent could cause the plan to be disqualified under certain circumstances.

Q. *How's that?*

A. Well, suppose we set the requirement at 2 per cent of salary and only the doctors employed by the corporation chose to participate on that basis. Then the I.R.S. could take the position that 2 per cent is too high a price to make employes pay for coverage; it could be ruled that the plan was discriminatory.

Q. *What if the I.R.S. doesn't disqualify the plan on that basis, yet the employe contribution requirement knocks out more than one of the employes, bringing the total of employes covered in our example down to, say, five?*

A. Then we have not satisfied the statutory requirement that our plan cover at least 80 per cent of the 70 per cent of employes who are eligible for the coverage.

Q. *And our plan is washed out?*

A. Not necessarily. If we satisfy either of the statutory requirements—either the 70 per cent test or the 80 per cent of 70 per cent test—we're home free. But if we don't, we still can apply to the I.R.S. district director for a special determination as to whether our plan is discriminatory or not.

Q. *You mean that he can approve a plan that does not meet statutory requirements?*

A. Yes. If he rules that we're justified in setting up the plan that we have, it's possible that he'll approve a plan that covers, say, 50 per cent of employes.

Q. *As a practical matter, though, won't most doctors who incorporate simply satisfy the 70 per cent rule—cover at least 70 per cent of their employes and leave it at that?*

A. Let's hope so. But I'll remind you that I set out to explain the outer limits of nondiscrimination, not necessarily to advocate their use.

Q. *What about a solo practitioner who's incorporating?*

A. He can have a plan for himself alone, if he has no employes—and that's often the case for a pathologist or anesthesiologist. If he has two employes—making three, himself included—he must cover all of them; 70 per cent of three is more than two, you see. But if there are a total of four employes, he may exclude one, because 70 per cent of four is less than three.

Q. *We've dealt with discrimination as it pertains to coverage of employes. Isn't there also a danger of discriminating in the way that contributions and benefits are allocated among employes who are covered?*

A. Yes, and I'll go into that. But it will help to bear in mind that when the Revenue Code speaks of contributions it's referring primarily to profit-sharing and money purchase retirement plans; when it speaks of benefits, it refers to pension plans which are geared to provide fixed payments on retirement.

Q. *In either type, then, the trick is to avoid showing favoritism to the corporation's officials–the doctors?*

A. Yes. And the easiest way to do that is to apportion contributions and benefits on the basis of employe earnings.

Q. *But doesn't that assure the doctors the lion's share?*

A. Of course; but they're contributing most to the fund, too. The important point is that the Revenue Code says we're not discriminating if we apportion contributions and benefits on the basis of compensation.

Q. *Would you spell out just how we do that?*

A. All right, here's an example. Suppose, for the sake of

simplicity, we have a corporation made up of one doctor and two office aides. This is our doctor who's been earning $50,000 a year and who's now cutting back to a salary of $40,000 in order to have $10,000 for a profit-sharing and pension plan. Each aide is eligible for coverage, we'll say, and each is earning an average of $6,000 a year.

Q. *So we have a total payroll of $52,000 and a contribution to the retirement plan of $10,000?*

A. Yes, and we want to apportion the contribution on the basis of salary. That means the doctor, with his salary of $40,000, will be entitled to $^{40}/_{52}$ of the total and each aide will be entitled to $^{6}/_{52}$. The doctor's share, then, is $7,692 and each aide's share should be about $1,150.

Q. *And we're talking here about a profit-sharing retirement plan?*

A. We're talking about a combined profit-sharing and money purchase plan for purposes of this example. But if we were setting up a defined benefit pension plan, we'd still apportion benefits on the basis of salary, to avoid any claims of discrimination. Age becomes an important factor in defined benefit plans, however.

Q. *How would we apply our example to the pension plan then?*

A. Under a defined benefit pension plan, we might provide for each employe to be paid, at retirement age, 50 per cent of his average salary for the previous five years.

Q. *Or 40 per cent, or 25 per cent?*

A. Yes, the percentage is what we decide it should be, but it must apply in the same way to all those covered. Let's figure it at 50 per cent. Then each aide at retirement would receive $3,000 a year from the corporation for the rest of her life, for example; we've said her average salary was $6,000.

The doctor's pension would come to $20,000 a year.

Q. *Benefits still are proportionate to salary?*

A. And nondiscriminatory. But now we must consider age. Let's assume that our incorporating doctor is 45, each aide is 25, and we've set 65 as retirement age. Then the corporation has 20 years to put enough money in a trust to fund the doctor's retirement benefits, but it has 40 years to put away enough to fund the girls' benefits. So we must apportion a much larger amount of each year's contribution to the doctor, because he has only half as much time remaining in the plan as the girls have.

Q. *You could even say, couldn't you, that the older the doctor and the younger his aides, the more suitable the defined benefit plan? Or that it's to the older doctor's advantage to hire young women . . .*

A. And to have such a plan rather than profit sharing. Of course, that assumes that he wants to maximize what he can contribute for himself.

Q. *There are other considerations, aren't there, in determining the type of retirement plan to use?*

A. Oh, yes. But the main one is: How much do you want to put into the plan? We've been discussing ways of putting in as little as possible and getting out as much as possible. But a basic point is that we can't put in more than 15 per cent of covered employees' salaries if we're going to have a profit-sharing plan alone and 25 per cent when combined with a money purchase plan up to a maximum dollar amount of $26,825 per year.

Q. *We're talking about before-tax dollars?*

A. Yes, and it's very important that doctors understand that. If I advise a doctor in the 50 per cent bracket to put $10,000 into his retirement plan, I'm actually asking him to live on only $5,000 less than he would have otherwise; he'd be paying half to the Government anyway.

Q. *What about vesting? Aren't there advantages to be had in the way that's handled?*

A. Yes, but vesting is primarily a means of holding employes you don't want to lose.

Q. *You require them to serve a certain length of time before they can claim benefits?*

A. That's right. We might say, for example, that the employe qualifies for inclusion in the plan after one year's employment. Then for each year of employment after the first, the aide can claim ownership of one-tenth of what's been put into the plan for her. She'd be fully vested after 10 years in the plan.

Q. *And if she left before becoming fully vested?*

A. Then she'd forfeit whatever was left in her account and hadn't yet been vested. If it's a profit-sharing plan, that forfeiture would increase proportionally the accounts of employes who remain. If it's a pension plan, the forfeiture would reduce subsequent contributions the corporation has to make to the plan. (However, if the corporation is making the maximum contribution, then forfeitures in the profit-sharing plan would be treated the same as in a pension plan.)

Q. *Then any advantage to the doctor from vesting . . .*

A. . . . would come from the way the vesting schedule was set up. It isn't difficult, that is, to design a schedule that encourages forfeitures.

Q. *We've talked pretty much about statutory provisions. Are there other ways to reach for minimum costs or maximum benefits?*

A. New ways are being tried all the time. One doctor corporation, for instance, tried to apportion the contribution on the basis of a point system that gave most weight to education and ran into trouble. (For details, see the box on pages 126-127.)

Q. *I've heard the term "integration with Social Security" used in relation to retirement plans. Is this a way to reduce costs?*

A. It's a way of either reducing costs or adding to benefits. Most professional corporations' plans should be integrated with Social Security. This permits the corporation to provide retirement benefits based only on wages in excess of those covered by Social Security. Lawyers setting up retirement plans have to understand all this, but for our purposes now, let's just say that integration with Social Security can reduce the cost of a plan about $225 a year for each employe. If you're covering five nondoctors, for example, integrating lets you reduce costs by more than $1,000 a year.

Q. *Getting back to those outer-limit devices for cutting down the cost of retirement plans: Do you approve of using any of them?*

A. Certainly; those provided for by statute. To reach beyond them, it seems to me, might be gambling dollars in the hope of winning pennies. It could result in the I.R.S. disqualifying your whole plan, and it could cost you some valued employes.

A PROFIT-SHARING PLAN THAT RAN INTO TROUBLE

How far can you go in reaching for minimum costs or maximum benefits under a profit-sharing plan without ending up guilty of discrimination? Before working out an elaborate plan of your own, better heed the sad experience of an Illinois professional corporation. A decision by a U.S. Court of Appeals found the doctors' plan showed discrimination over a period of three years and opened the way to a formidable financial loss now that it has been disqualified.

When Dr. Max Goldenberg, an East St. Louis, Ill., internist, set up a profit-sharing plan for his incorporated clinic, there were no guidelines on what sort of plan might be approved or disapproved. His clinic created a plan and a trust that called for a contribution for each eligible employe of 5 per cent of total compensation. Eligibility depended upon three years with the clinic or with the partnership that preceded it.

But in the first year, the plan didn't seem to be doing the job intended, Goldenberg says. Besides being costly, it didn't provide the fringe-benefit incentive to keep employes with the clinic or to inspire them to become more valuable employes as time went by. The area in which the clinic operates, Goldenberg points out, is a low-opportunity section of East St. Louis and poses a problem in attracting and holding both doctors and other staffers.

To help combat that problem, Goldenberg continues, a new profit-sharing plan was worked out and put into effect in three years after he first incorporated. Under that plan, each participating employe was assigned points for length of service—one point for each year of service up to a maximum of five. Points were also assigned for experience and for job-related education. To arrive at an allocation figure for each employe, his education and training points were totaled and the sum multiplied by his service points. Thus, Dr. Goldenberg's formula produced an allocation of 20 per cent of his compensation, 12 per cent for the doctor with the next highest allocation, and 2 per cent for the doctor with the lowest allocation. The clinic's business manager and staff received allocations ranging from 7½ per cent to 2 per cent.

Before the elaborate formula was put into effect, Goldenberg wrote the I.R.S. "What we wanted would now be called a letter of determination, a ruling telling us our plan was qualified," says Goldenberg, "or at least letting us know we might be headed for trouble. We received no answer at all and went ahead." "When the I.R.S. responded, it didn't answer our basic question as to whether our plan qualified," Goldenberg says. "About all it did do was set us to worrying about what sort of guidelines we could follow if there were such things as guidelines, and if the I.R.S. recognized such an animal as a professional corporation." The doctor's worry coincided with increasing publicity about the guidelines Keogh plans could be expected to follow.

So, taking its cue from approved Keogh plans, the clinic dropped the complex formula and went back to its former 5 per cent allocation of employes' compensation, based on seniority. Then the I.R.S. ruled that the old formula wasn't qualified and that the funds paid into it were therefore taxable. Clinic employes sued the U.S. for refund of the taxes. But the I.R.S. lost in a district court decision, which found the formula plan wasn't discriminatory. The higher paid employes, doctors, justifiably drew a greater percentage of the profits, because they contributed more to the earnings and resulting profits, the district court held. But the U.S. Court of Appeals for the Seventh Circuit overruled that decision with a finding that pretty well puts the lid on profit-sharing plans that attempt to set up greatly differing rates of allocation among employes.

Sweeping aside arguments that Goldenberg had designed the formula to create a more effective medical organization, the court said that the plan discriminated in favor of the officers and highly compensated employes. "It seems to us," the court ruled, "that a plan must be deemed to discriminate where the ratio of allocation to compensation is substantially higher for highly compensated employes than for others."

13 Choosing corporate fringes that won't break you

As every incorporated doctor knows, providing fringe benefits for the office staff can be a major expense. In fact, they can be so expensive that just the prospect of paying them may very well have led you to reject the whole idea of incorporation. But here's a surprise: They needn't be backbreaking at all.

What you may not have realized is that you have a wide variety of fringe-benefit options available. How you pick and choose among them will have a dramatic effect on the amount you have to lay out each year. At one extreme, fringe-benefit costs could boost your payroll expense by about a third; at the other, they'd come to just a tiny fraction. As the illustrations below show, fringe benefits for a payroll of $15,000 can range from almost $5,000 to as little as $500. True, the expense is tax-deductible, but it still costs you money. That's one good reason you should know whether what you're spending provides benefits that are deluxe, standard, or minimal.

Deluxe benefits. If your pension and profit-sharing plans provide for contributions at a flat rate of 25 per cent of salaries for all employes, you're committed to a very expensive fringe-benefit package. If, in addition, those contributions vest immediately, so that all corporate employes can take all their retirement-plan money with them whenever they leave, then there's no detour off the expensive route. Simple math shows that you've increased your payroll costs by 25 cent.

Your health and disability benefits also may be overblown if you provide basic medical and hospital insurance and major-medical coverage. Another expensive setup is to

---

TYPICAL FRINGE-BENEFIT COSTS FOR A $15,000 PAYROLL

As this chapter explains, the amount you can spend on corporate fringe benefits for your employes ranges from almost nothing to a burdensome load. Benefits besides those shown here would have only a marginal effect on total cost.

	Deluxe	Standard	Minimal
Retirement Plans	$3,750	$1,100	$500
Disability and Health Payments	$1,200	$ 450	0
Life Insurance	$ 20	$ 8	0
Total	$4,970	$1,558	$500

specify simply that every employe is entitled to reimbursement for medical expenses and disability insurance costs up to a flat amount of salary, say 8 per cent. For a payroll of $15,000, either of those arrangements could cost about $1,200 a year, adding a significant percentage to your payroll expenses.

As for group life insurance, the third major corporate fringe benefit, new programs for small groups have been marketed so the cost is cheap no matter how you arrange it. Say you have two young women on your staff, who make a total of $15,000 a year. You can buy life insurance covering them for the full amount of their earnings for about $25 a year. Still, it may be an indication that you've chosen a deluxe program when you'd really be happier providing somewhat less.

Standard benefits. One of the simplest ways to cut down the cost of retirement-plan contributions, the most expensive corporate fringe benefit, is to integrate your plans with Social Security. "Integration" is a fancy way of saying that you can coordinate the contributions to the plans your corporation voluntarily sets up with the ones you must make to the Government's retirement plan. You do that by building the corporation's plans on top of Social Security and paying for benefits based only on wages in excess of the amount that the Government covers. That move alone could drastically cut the costs of your pension and profit-sharing plan.

From that point on, the choices you make may very well be dictated by circumstances. With a schedule of vesting that allows a departing employe to take away only a certain portion of his money in the pension and profit-sharing accounts—based on length of service—there's a good chance that a good bit of the money you contribute for employes will remain with you through forfeitures. (See previous chapter for details.)

Until recently, there was a problem with that because there was no uniform Internal Revenue Service policy on vesting. That's been changed now, though. As a result, many corporations have much shorter vesting schedules in their pension and profit-sharing plans than the I.R.S. requires. Whether you should stretch out vesting as long as you're allowed to is a matter that we'll take up later on in this chapter.

If you're over 50, you should consider a pension plan in which contributions are set to provide a specific benefit rather than one based on contributions as a percentage of salaries. For example, this type of benefit-funded plan might specify that at age 65 an employe will receive retirement pay equal to, say, 50 per cent of average salary for the previous five years. (Social Security benefits can be subtracted from these payments.) If you're 55, and the average age of the staff is 30, it stands to reason that the corporation will have to put away a much greater amount of each year's contribution to provide your pension than it will for the others. That's because there's more time to build up their pension funds.

If you have four or more employes in the corporation, then you may be able to take advantage of another cost-cutting device—designing pension and profit-sharing plans so that not all employes are included.

Another place to prune excessive fringe-benefit costs is in corporate health and disability plans. There's no requirement that you must provide the same benefits to all employes. For example, you could provide a plan that reimburses employes for expenses of medical bills and health and disability insurance on a percentage scale of, say, 2 per cent of the first $5,000 of earnings, 5 per cent of the next, and 10 per cent on everything over that. Another way might be to have a plan that provides basic hospitalization and medical insurance for the office staff, while giving the doctors major-medical and disability coverage in addition to that. Either way, you could cut this benefit down to about a third of the cost of the deluxe route.

If you set life insurance coverage according to employment classifications—so much for receptionists, so much for technicians, and so on—you can probably pay less than if you provide a flat amount geared to earnings. Set the top scale at $50,000, though. That's the maximum tax-deductible amount and what you want for yourself. Either way, however, the cost is so low as not to matter—unless you have a large staff or older employes on the payroll.

Minimal benefits. It's possible to cut the costs of a corporate fringe program down to almost nothing, but it's risky and probably poor employe relations to boot. Basically, to use this approach, you take full advantage of all the cost-cutting techniques already mentioned, and you don't give your employes any coverage for medical and disability expenses.

The danger of cutting back fringe benefits too far is that you could run afoul of I.R.S. rules that might disqualify your retirement plans. For example, if you have a vesting schedule that holds off benefits for 10 years or so, and the turnover in your office is so high that none of the staff ever get any benefits, an agent could charge that your plan is discriminatory in operation and revoke I.R.S. approval.

The situation with medical and disability benefits is slightly different. The law is in a state of flux now as the courts decide which plans are adequate and which aren't. To be safe, you should make sure that all full-time employes are covered to some extent.

That's the overview of what the three main approaches to a fringe-benefit program mean in terms of cost. If you've shied away from incorporation because it seemed too expensive, you may want to consider it again. If you incorporated and are now dissatisfied with the cost of existing fringes, then you should consider cutting back on them.

The main job in cutting back will be making sure your retirement plan still qualifies for I.R.S. approval. To make such a change, you'll also have to vest the amounts that have already been deposited in employes' accounts—a relatively small price to pay for getting things as you want them from here on. If you're reducing health and disability benefits, it takes only a simple amendment to your plans. You'll still have to explain the cuts to your employes, of course. And, as you'll see in the next chapter, there's one fringe benefit you don't even have to provide your employes.

EVEN CHEAPER THAN KEOGH? YOU BET!

Incorporated physicians are presented with a wide range of cost choices in providing fringe benefits for their office staffs. In fact, most doctors would be amazed to find that some fringe-benefit plans can cost even less than under Keogh.

For example, take an unincorporated doctor netting $50,000 with a staff earning $15,000 a year. To get the full $7,500 into his own Keogh plan, it would cost that doctor $2,250 a year for his employes—substantially more than even the standard corporate fringe-benefit route, as shown on page 130.

4 AN EXTRA CORPORATE RETIREMENT PLAN JUST FOR YOU

Despite all the talk about retirement plans, you probably haven't heard of a special kind—one that has the unusual advantage of not being under the thumb of the Internal Revenue Service. Available to doctors in incorporated groups, this type is known as a nonqualified retirement plan. (Solo doctors may simply accumulate profits. For details, see the box on pages 140-141.) Under its provisions, you don't have to include the office staff—in fact, you don't even have to include all the doctors in your group.

You can set the benefits any way you like, based on service with the corporation, service prior to the formation of the corporation, or a combination of the two. And the terms can be as generous as you alone or you and your colleagues together can afford. To finance benefits, you can set up a special fund out of current income, or you can pay them out of future income. Admittedly, that can be a problem as will be explained below. What's important is that a nonqualified plan can serve you well if:

You can get along with less now in return for more retirement pay. Take a three-man partnership with one older man and two younger ones. The two younger men had been reluctant to incorporate because they needed as much current income as possible to meet their family obligations. The older man's problem was to build his assets as quickly as possible in the few years he had left before retirement.

The extra retirement plan meshed easily with their needs. As a partnership, they'd been splitting income equally. After they incorporated, the older man dropped his salary $5,000, and the other two split the $5,000 between them. When the senior doctor retires, he has a special contract with the corporation to pay him $5,000 a year—the money the others are getting now—until he's even.

This way, all three are happy: The younger men have the advantage of the extra income now, and the older one gets his share back when he's in a lower tax bracket.

Such an arrangement is not difficult to set up. It can simply be included as a section in the employment contract, according to Atlanta attorney Harry V. Lamon Jr.

While that doctor's retirement payments are guaranteed by contract, the fact is that he's still taking a chance. For instance, if his colleagues decided to break up the corporation after he left it, he'd have no one to look to for the money. That's one of the risks in an unfunded plan.

One doctor I know doesn't have to worry about that possibility. He, too, is in a three-man group and has taken a salary cut in order to get more money later. However, instead of having the money paid out currently to the other doctors, it's being put into a special account where it will be available after he retires—no matter what the other doctors decide. This type of arrangement is called a funded plan.

You arrange for new doctors to make your retirement payments as part of the buy-in. You can set up a plan that won't require you to take any cut in current earnings if the payments come out of corporate earnings after you retire. The effect of that is to put the burden on new doctors who join the group.

Can you get doctors to join a group if they know they're going to have this kind of future call on their earnings? Yes, if you can convince them that the retirement payments they'll be paying out are no different than payments that used to be routinely made for goodwill—only easier to take. In addition, it can be pointed out that retirement benefits are tax-deductible to those paying them, and they'll come in the future when the new doctors will be better able to afford them. These points should make it easier to bargain with the new men.

Even so, some groups may find it hard to present convincing arguments. In that case, there's another way to turn retirement payments into an attraction. Let's back up a bit to understand better how this plan works.

In the usual situation, a new man is paid less than he earns currently, with the difference going to the senior doctors. In turn, the younger man gets shares in the existing accounts receivable, so everything works out in time.

But there's one drawback. The younger man probably has bigger obligations, including paying off the loans he took to get through school. He needs more now—not later—and with this type of retirement payments setup, the group can pay him more at first. Instead of getting less than he earns, as would usually be the case, he gets exactly what he produces.

Things even out when he makes payments later on when the older men retire.

By that time, the new man will have hit his stride and be in a better position to pay the money. Then, too, the older men are probably earning less in retirement, so they have to pay less taxes than if they'd gotten the money while they were working. This should be clearly spelled out in the contract, though, so nobody forgets the earlier break.

What about the accounts receivable? Until all the retirement benefits have been paid, the younger man has no claim on them. That gives the older man security for payment in case the younger man leaves prior to the senior's retirement.

You want a payoff for extra services. Say you're the founder of a practice that's grown to a fair-size group. You feel that the newer men are now benefiting from your hard work in the years when they weren't even there and that you should get something for it. Well, you can bet that the younger men won't agree if it involves shelling out money after you're gone.

If you feel you have such a claim on the corporation's earnings, the best time to make it is when the group is incorporating. That's when all the relationships in the partnership agreement are subject to negotiation. If you can't get the group to agree to full payments, it may be possible to work out a plan that's partially funded with the money you slice off your salary now and the rest from payments out of profits later. In effect, you'd be sharing the cost of your extra pension with the men who remain.

If you decide to set up a nonqualified retirement plan, one of your key decisions will be whether to fund it by setting aside corporate earnings or by paying benefits out of future earnings. If your plan is funded, the corporation will have to pay tax on the money each year as it's set aside, and then you'll have to pay tax on it again later when you get it.

On the other hand, funds that are set aside can be invested, and if the earnings come from dividends of other corporations, then they're practically tax-free. What's more, you're sure that the money will be there when you want it.

One detail to remember: In a funded plan, there's a legal requirement that you can't have an absolute right to the money. If you do, then you're taxed on it right away instead of later on when you retire. To handle that requirement, you can simply have a provision requiring you to forfeit payments if you compete with the group after you leave.

If you set up an unfunded plan where the retirement payments will come out of future earnings, it's best to key them to gross income, according to Marvin Kamensky, a Chicago attorney who's set up many such plans. For a smaller group, Kamensky says you might set payments as high as 4 or 5 per cent of the group's gross. For a larger group, they'd be scaled down to as little as one-half of 1 per cent of gross. To avoid an open-ended deal, you should set a limit on the total to be paid.

The payments would continue according to the way you set up the plan. For example, you might say that a man would get payments for one month for each year he was with the corporation and for one month for each two years he was with the practice prior to the formation of the corporation. If a doctor had 14 years with the practice before the corporation and 10 afterwards, then he'd get payments for 17 months. If the group grossed $40,000 a month, and payments were set at 5 per cent, he'd get $2,000 a month for 17 months—a total of $34,000.

Kamensky also favors putting a dollar limit on monthly payments—as a convenience to the corporation rather than a ceiling on the doctor's benefits. In such a case, if the gross grows to a point where the payments would be over the limit, they're simply paid out later.

For example, take that plan that's geared to pay $2,000 monthly. Let's say it has a limit of $2,500 on the monthly

---

NOW IT MAY PAY TO ACCUMULATE CORPORATE PROFITS

Until recently, many solo and small multispecialty professional corporations have been advised to budget salaries and other costs so that the total comes as close as possible to practice receipts. The idea in leaving as little corporate net profit as possible was based on the fact that the I.R.S. usually held that profits not paid as dividends—and taxed twice—were subject to a 70 per cent penalty tax.

However, the I.R.S. has reversed itself with a ruling (Rev. Rul. 75-67) that exempts almost all professional corporations from the penalty tax. A corporation still has to pay some tax on its profit, but at the modest rate of 20 per cent on the first $25,000 and 22 per cent on the next $25,000. Presumably, that's a lot lower than the tax levied in your personal bracket. After the corporation pays its taxes, it can invest what's left in dividend-paying stock, paying only 3 per cent tax on dividends.

Accumulating corporate funds in this way may be just the ticket for you if you'll have to cut back on contributions to your retirement plans because of the limitations of the Pension Reform Act of 1974. Whether or not you're crimped by that, it would be a good idea to look into the new profit-accumulation picture to see if there'd be income tax or future estate tax advantages.

Commenting on the opportunities afforded by the special tax breaks on corporate income, Alan S. Finger, an attorney with payout and that the gross in some months comes to $55,000. At 5 per cent, the retired M.D. would be entitled to $2,750, but that would be $250 above the ceiling. Would he lose it? Not at all. It could be credited to his account and paid out after the 17-month schedule of benefits ended or given him in a month when the gross dropped to a point where the payment would be below the ceiling.

---

the Chicago firm of Katten, Muchin, Gitles, Zavis, Pearl and Galler, points out the key ground rules.

If the money stays in the corporation until you retire, you'll be taxed at a favorable capital gains rate. But the corporate taxes and the final capital gains tax may be little more than the levy on benefits from a tax-sheltered retirement plan.

Under the present law, there will be no capital gains tax if you die before you retire and leave corporate assets as part of your estate. However, there will be an estate tax. You'll recall that retirement money is exempt from estate tax but is subject to income tax.

Thus, if you divert some of the money you might put into your retirement plan and hold it in the corporation, you may be able to reduce the over-all tax bite on your estate. You'd be aiming to shift money from a high income tax bracket to a lower estate tax bracket.

Those are the ground rules for solos. Although the new I.R.S. ruling also exempts small multispecialty corporations from the penalty tax on retained earnings, it would be impractical for them to use their profits as solos would.

There's a practical limit on how much you should accumulate, though. If you build up more than $150,000 in corporate accumulated profits, then the corporation may be liable for a special tax of 27½ per cent on the next $100,000.

"Even if such a strategy seems worthwhile, get your advisers to check out the dollars and cents of your situation before you let corporate profits build up," Finger cautions.

15 HOW A CORPORATION CAN SLASH YOUR ESTATE TAXES

Whether you're incorporated or not, you've probably heard all about the amount of income tax a professional corporation can save you. Admittedly, the prospect of saving money on income taxes had a way of turning on most people pretty quickly, but that's only half the story: There often are even greater corporate gains to be made in estate tax savings. So it will pay you to become familiar with the pointers outlined here.

If you haven't yet incorporated, some additional facts about the advantages can help you make up your mind. If you've already incorporated, you could discover that you're letting half of the estate tax benefits of a professional corporation slip through your fingers. In that event, don't waste any more time. What you do could mean a difference of tens of thousands of dollars for your heirs. (The accompanying table pinpoints specific dollar savings for a typical case.)

The extent of those potential savings was brought home to me recently in discussions with advisers specializing in professional corporations in a cross section of areas across the country. Here is a distillation of their advice.

Give up ownership of corporation-paid group-term life insurance. It's easy to overlook life insurance your corporation has taken out on you—even if you've thought about the estate tax problem. One reason is that the premiums are paid out as a business expense, so the money doesn't seem to

HOW PROPER ESTATE PLANNING PAYS OFF

The example below shows the dramatic Federal estate tax savings possible for a doctor who decided to pull out all the stops in planning his estate. The figures cited take into account $200,000 of assets in addition to the ones shown and assume that the doctor would have a will leaving half of his estate to his wife outright. The other half would go into a trust paying her income for life, with the principal thereafter going to the children.

ASSET AND AMOUNT
Group insurance—$50,000
Employe death benefit—$5,000
Furniture and equipment—$25,000
Pension plan—200,000
Corporate stock—$5,000
Accounts receivable—$35,000
Nonqualified pension plan—$10,000

come out of your pocket. When your family collects the proceeds, though, Uncle Sam isn't going to forget. If you've named your wife as the beneficiary of your corporate policies, half of the proceeds will be taxed at your death. And if you've planned poorly, the Government could tax what's left of that half all over again and the other half, too, when your wife dies later on. From the typical $50,000 coverage, your children could thus end up with very little of the original proceeds.

WRONG WAY	RIGHT WAY	SAVINGS[1]
Left outright	Left in trust to wife, then to children	$ 12,200
None provided	Payment provided	700
Owned by corporation	Owned separately by trust	7,000
Left outright to wife (or other beneficiary)	Left in trust to wife, then to children	60,100
Insurance-funded buyout increasing value to $55,000	No insurance in buyout, but additional group term left with other insurance	15,100[2]
Paid out by corporation	Kept by corporation, but insurance paid instead	10,850[2]
Left outright to wife	Left in trust for wife, then to children	3,100[2]
	Total Savings	**$109,050**

[1]*These figures represent the taxes that would otherwise have been paid at the death of the doctor and/or his wife.*
[2]*These savings available only to doctors in incorporated groups.*

A simple method of dealing with the problem was chosen by a doctor I recently talked with: He made his wife the owner of the policy. That potentially eliminates estate tax liability on the insurance at the doctor's death, but the proceeds still would be taxed at his wife's death.

Attorney Marvin Kamensky suggests a way around that by setting up an irrevocable insurance trust. It can provide that the wife will get the trust income as long as she lives, and she can withdraw the principal, too, if she needs it. That way, she gets just as much out of the insurance as if it had come right into her hands. And of course, when the wife dies, the trust funds go to the children, who escape having to pay the estate tax that would otherwise fall due.

While Kamensky indicates that irrevocable trusts of this type should not be set up without considerable thought, they can effect substantial tax savings.

Have a $5,000 death-benefit clause in your employment contract. The mere inclusion of such a provision exempts the payment from both estate and income taxes, yet many employment contracts don't have it, says New York City attorney Leonard Bailin. The irony is that a death-benefit clause doesn't have to cost the corporation a cent. If you're in an incorporated group, the corporation can simply provide that the $5,000 will be deducted from your other benefits; if you're solo, the $5,000 can be automatic.

Keep corporate assets as lean as possible. If you separate ownership of equipment and furnishings from the corporation, it's possible to give them away and bypass estate taxes and probate costs as well. If the corporation owns the assets, your family will be penalized. Their value will be added to the value of the corporate stock and taxed as part of your estate.

The easy way to dispose of corporate assets is to give them to your wife, if you're solo, or to set up a separate partnership if you're in a group and give away your interest in the equipment partnership.

A still better way is to set up an equipment trust with your children as the beneficiaries. That way, the corporation can pay rent for the equipment and furniture, and those payments will count as the children's trust income. Since they're probably paying little or no tax, there'll be an income tax saving now as well as an estate tax saving later on. Here's how this plan might work out:

You set up an equipment trust for your children, contributing $50,000 worth of assets to it that you had in your medical practice. The corporation pays the trust a rental of $5,000 a year—money that would otherwise have been paid out largely to the doctor and taxed in your high bracket. Because your children have no other income, they pay no tax at all, so there's a saving of about $2,000 a year in Federal income tax. The money is used to pay for private school education, camp, and other extras. (It's better for the trust income to be used for luxuries. If it's used for items you're required to furnish, the I.R.S. would make you pay tax on it.) If you die before you retire, the assets in the trust will be exempt from estate tax and probate costs.

Caution: You have to set up the rental payments in an "arms-length" transaction. That means having a truly independent trustee; also, the rent that the corporation and the trustee agree on has to be reasonable. And unless your share of the corporation's assets are worth a substantial amount—at least $25,000, say—it won't pay to go to the expense and bother of setting up an equipment trust.

Check the beneficiary of your pension and profit-sharing

plans. While your primary motive in putting money away is probably to build up assets for retirement, remember that there's an important estate tax advantage that's easily overlooked. If you should die before you retire, the money in your pension and profit-sharing plans is exempt from estate tax, provided it's paid to a named beneficiary—either an individual or a trust. So it's important to make sure that you've executed a beneficiary designation form. That will keep the tax men away if something happens to you.

You can score a double play on the I.R.S. if you set up a trust to receive your retirement funds in the event that you die before retirement. The one a New Jersey internist recently had his lawyer form provides that any money in it shall be invested, with the income paid to the doctor's wife as long as she lives. If that isn't enough to support her comfortably, then the trustee has the right to dip into principal. Upon the wife's death, the money will be paid to her children. And not one dime will go to the Government in estate taxes.

Leif C. Beck, a management consultant in Bala Cynwyd, Pa., adds a caution here: There should be a specific prohibition against the trust's using any of the money from the pension and profit-sharing plans for payment of estate tax or the claims of the estate's creditors. Even the possibility that the money could be used in that way could result in making it taxable in your estate, Beck warns.

So far, the moves we've discussed will work for all incorporated doctors, whether solo or in a group. If you're in a group, though, consider the following additional steps.

Avoid an insurance-funded stock-purchase agreement. There are advantages to having insurance to provide the funds for buying up a departed doctor's share of the stock:

The corporation pays no tax on the proceeds it gets and simply hands over the money to the family of the deceased doctor; and the heirs thus may end up with thousands more than the stock was worth if the doctor had sold it to his colleagues while he lived. The big drawback, however, is that family members pay estate tax on every cent of the money they get under an insurance-funded agreement.

It's better to have the corporation pay your heirs exactly what the stock is worth—normally the depreciated value of the assets plus any cash on hand at the date the stock is evaluated. If you decide you want an additional death benefit, then James D. Vaughan, a Ridgewood, N.J., pension planner, recommends that you establish a group-term insurance program. That way, ownership of the insurance can be transferred so there's no estate tax to pay.

But make sure there's no connection between the term

SMOOTHING THE WAY FOR A SOLO CORPORATION

If you're the only shareholder in your corporation, you should take care to check a few estate-related details now. If you haven't taken care of them, your family could have extra difficulties if you die before winding up practice. Attorney Alan Finger says that you should make sure your wife or some other person besides yourself has the authority to sign corporate checks. You should also have a second person act with you as trustee of your pension and profit-sharing plans. And if state law permits, you should have your wife or another person as an officer in your corporation. With an additional person having the authority to act in your place, he or she could take over at your death. Without that, everything could be held up until a probate judge decided to permit your executor to take over.

insurance and the stock. If the I.R.S. smells that the benefits are in lieu of money for the stock, it'll be taxed, no matter what. It's also true that if the face value of the insurance exceeds $50,000, then you'll have to pay a small amount of income tax on it each year. But the estate tax advantage your family would receive should outweigh that drawback.

Protect accounts receivable from estate tax. The amounts due from patients are often the most substantial part of a medical practice's assets, and their handling can be tricky for the estate of a doctor in an incorporated group. If they're

---

WHO'D PAY OUT YOUR RETIREMENT FUNDS IF YOU DIED?

If you're in a one-man corporation, and you're also the trustee of the retirement plan, there could be trouble—unless you plan now. When management consultant Edward G. Marquis of Columbus, Ohio, was killed in a plane crash, many of his professional corporation clients had a special loss. He'd been the trustee of over 100 corporate pension and profit-sharing plans, and it was necessary to get a replacement. Otherwise, there'd be no one authorized to run the plans or disburse the funds.

The Marquis case brings into focus the entire problem of succession of trustees in a corporate retirement plan. It's a problem that you may likely have overlooked.

In this case, the doctors didn't have much trouble getting a new trustee. They were notified that Marquis's associates at Professional Practice Management would be willing to serve as successors. The transfer was accomplished by each corporation when its board of directors voted for a new trustee.

The transition might be more troublesome if you're in a one-man corporation and serve as the trustee and the sole director.

counted as part of the corporate assets, they jack up the price of the stock. And since the stock has to be bought with after-tax dollars, it's more difficult to sell when the receivables are included. So receivables are usually handled sepa rately from stocks.

When a doctor leaves a corporation, he (or his heirs) sells his stock for its nominal value, and the accounts receivable are paid out as severance pay. Trouble is, in that form, the money is subject to estate tax and income tax as well.

It's possible to avoid both those taxes by arranging for the

If something happened to you, there'd be no director to approve the choice of a new trustee. Someone would have to get the authority to appoint a new director, and he in turn would then name the new trustee. Meanwhile, if the trust funds were invested in securities, they might go down the drain, and nobody could make a move to save them for your heirs.

A co-trustee could be the answer, but not if it's your wife. That's because if you were both killed in an accident, there'd be no one to manage the trust, just the same as if you alone had been the trustee.

At the death of the doctor in a one-man corporation, an executor would usually have to be appointed before a new trustee could be named. Thus, any problem with probate could spill over to the retirement plan and extend the hiatus between trustees.

To avoid the problem of a trustee-less trust, many lawyers recommend that you appoint an alternate trustee to take over in case something happens to the trustee of the retirement plan. That would provide continuity of management and would assure your heirs of getting what's coming to them with the least possible delay. So if you're the trustee of your plan, better check with your lawyer to see if some such move is indicated in your case.

family to get the proceeds of an insurance policy tacked onto the group coverage instead of an additional payment from the corporation. Here again the doctor will have to pay a small amount of income tax each year on the money the corporation pays for coverage in excess of $50,000, but it's a small price compared to the benefits for his heirs.

Since insurance can be pretty expensive for older doctors, and some income tax must be paid on premiums spent for coverage in excess of $50,000, there's a practical limit on how far you can work this. But you'll probably want to check it out.

Leave extra corporate benefits in trust. If you have a non-qualified pension plan—one that includes the right to payments from the corporation after you leave—there's no way to avoid taxation on the payments to your estate. If you're setting up a trust anyway, though, you can have the benefits paid to that trust, so there won't be a second tax when your beneficiary dies.

There you have the broad outlines of the kind of plan you should be thinking about if you're in a professional corporation. As you can see from the table on page 144, the savings can be enormous. Of course, you'll have to check with your individual advisers on what's best for you and what can be done in your particular case. Even if you decide not to change things radically, you're in a better planning position knowing what could happen to your practice assets if you don't make it to retirement.

16 don't be oversold on corporate life insurance

If you're thinking of incorporating or already have incorporated, life insurance salesmen are probably urging you to buy more coverage for your corporate retirement plan. But you'd better examine the pros and cons carefully before being talked into this action. The amount of insurance the salesman advocates may be more than you need.

The proportion of annual contributions to corporate retirement funds that may be used to purchase life insurance is generally limited by law. In line with this, many insurance agents urge their doctor-clients to buy the legal maximum. They are often successful because they employ several persuasive arguments based on this thesis: The more coverage you can build into your retirement fund, the better. Here are the major points they make—along with some counterarguments.

▶*The premiums are tax-deductible to the corporation, so you get a bargain rate.*

True—but you might not need a good part of what that bargain rate would buy. Probably a good many of your insurance needs have already been taken care of by policies you've bought outside your retirement plan. Be very wary of proposals that you surrender your old policies and buy new ones or that you transfer your present coverage into the retirement plan. Attempting to do so can get you into legal or financial difficulties.

▶*The death benefit of any life insurance that's part of your retirement fund won't be included in your estate for Federal tax purposes.*

This is not as strong an argument as it might seem. The same result could be attained by making your wife (or an irrevocable trust) the owner of the policies—if that fits in with your estate plan. A big advantage of making an irrevocable trust the owner of insurance policies is that the death benefit escapes taxation at both your death and your wife's.

▶*Present annuity rates are guaranteed at retirement.*

Despite the ever-increasing life expectancy, the reason recent changes in annuity rates have been on the plus side is that insurance companies have achieved high earnings and effective cost control. Thus it may be that the money you put into insurance now with the option of converting to an annuity at retirement will not necessarily bring in a larger income than an annuity you could buy for the same amount when you retire.

▶*Your equity in an insurance policy is guaranteed, which makes it a very sound investment.*

But your equity is also pretty well guaranteed in high-grade bonds, savings accounts, and various forms of Government bills. And at present they offer considerably higher yields than insurance policies.

▶*Life insurance in your retirement fund gives an immediate and substantial benefit in case of death.*

Yes, but an immediate death benefit can also be established inexpensively outside the fund through group life insurance—with the premiums tax-deductible to the corporation.

The physician in a split-funded retirement plan will usually either convert the fund to an annuity at retirement time or else take it in a lump sum. Therefore I feel that the insurance in such a plan should be considered only as coverage for needs that may be expected to exist up to retirement time. For a typical physician, such needs may well include funds for:

His children's general support and education. By the time he retires, the children presumably will be on their own.

Home mortgage payments. The mortgage usually will be paid off by the time he retires.

Business loans, including mortgages on commercial real estate. And these, too, will probably be fully amortized when he retires.

To sum up, putting a moderate amount of corporate retirement-plan contributions into an ordinary life policy is probably a good idea—so long as the coverage is intended for specific needs that will no longer exist once you reach retirement age.

17 THE I.R.S. SETS DOCTOR CORPORATIONS STRAIGHT

It's some years now since the Internal Revenue Service announced that it would recognize professional corporations formed pursuant to state law. That ruling ended litigation over the question of whether professionals could gain "corporateness" and legitimatized professional corporations. But the I.R.S. also ruled that it still reserves the right to "conclude differently in cases reflecting special circumstances." That has raised the spectre of additional troubles. Even without any additional threat, a professional corporation should be very circumspect.

Obviously, professional corporations are being watched, though precisely what they're going to be watched for may vary with the circumstances. To find out, Medical Economics arranged to interview K. Martin Worthy, when he was the I.R.S. chief counsel. In that role, he was in a key position to interpret the laws and regulations on professional corporations. Here are Worthy's frank answers to questions posed by Medical Economics.

Q. *Doctors and some of their tax advisers have been concerned about the possibility that professional corporations will be targets for audit. Is there any basis for that?*

A. Since the I.R.S. audits a higher percentage of corporate returns than individual ones, a doctor does increase his chance of being audited when he incorporates. But I know of no plan to make more intensive audits of professional corporations than of any other corporations.

Q. *Many doctors who practice as individuals or in partnership like to handle their own tax audits. Will they still be able to do that after they incorporate?*

A. Not generally. A corporation has many problems that an individual doesn't have. One of the reasons for incorporating in the first place is to get the advantages of a corporate retirement plan. Inevitably, such a plan introduces new complexities into the taxpayer's return and increases the chances for error.

Q. *When a corporate return is selected for audit, will the doctor-shareholder's individual return be checked over too?*

A. Frequently.

Q. *In addition to the retirement plan, what other things is an I.R.S. auditor likely to check when he reviews a corporation's tax return?*

A. How it operates. It's not enough to get the charter and then put it up on the shelf and continue to operate as before. In other words, to be recognized as a corporation, professionals—or anyone for that matter—must not only organize the corporation properly, they must operate it as one, too.

Q. *Is management by a board of directors important as an*

indication that a professional corporation is really operating in corporate form?

A. Certainly. Although there may be some states that permit a one-man corporation to operate without a board of directors, in the overwhelming majority of cases, it's required. The board should have a regular time and place for its meetings and should meet at those times and places. If there are members of the board who aren't actively employed by the corporation, as is permissible under the laws of some states, they should still take an interest in the affairs of the corporation. They shouldn't be mere dummies. The board must be duly elected and must actually conduct the business affairs of the corporation.

Q. *What sort of corporate business affairs?*

A. While the individual state statutes will control the specifics, the board should ordinarily set the salaries and bonuses of the officers, for example.

Q. *Must the board pass on the salaries of the nonprofessionals, too?*

A. No. That authority could be delegated to one of the corporation's officers or the business manager. I might add that, in the case of a large clinic—one with 50 professionals, for example—the board could also delegate the responsibility for setting the compensation of all but the major officers.

Q. *What about the board's role in the retirement plan?*

A. Certainly the plan itself would have to be approved by the board. It would also have to pass on any changes. And if the plan permitted flexibility—as in a profit-sharing plan with a sliding scale of contributions depending on the corporation's profits each year—then the board would have to vote on that, too.

Q. *What about major expenditures—say, the purchase of*

an X-ray machine, for example?

A. That would have to be judged in context of the size of the corporation. I wouldn't expect the board of the Mayo Clinic to vote on whether to buy an X-ray machine. On the other hand, that might be a very important expenditure for a one-man or two-man corporation. In general, where there's a doubt on whether the board of directors should act or not, I'd say it doesn't hurt to take a vote. Where a major expenditure is linked with a change of operations, as in the construction of a new building to house the medical corporation, the board should always pass on it.

Q. *So far, we've been talking about the management of the corporation. What will a tax auditor look for in the actual running of the medical practice?*

A. One of the most important questions is whom patients are dealing with. What is the contractual relationship? Is the patient employing Dr. Smith or is he employing the Smith, Jones, and Brown Corporation? It's vitally important that the professional corporation conduct itself so that the patients know they're dealing with a corporation—even though the doctors will continue to provide the medical services.

The implications of those questions are highly technical, but in general terms, if we find that the patients are really dealing with the doctors as individuals, the corporation is in effect a sham. That's what a court ruled in one case. (For details, see box on page 48.) Even if the corporation stands up, it still may be possible to allocate the income to the individual doctor.

Q. *What procedure would you recommend to make sure patients know they're dealing with a corporation?*

A. First, all patients should be notified in writing that a

corporation has been formed. Then, the corporation's name should be on all bills and correspondence, and those bills and letters should go out in the name of the corporation. Prescriptions should be written in the corporate name although the individual doctor will probably have to sign them.

Q. *What about the internal operations of the professional corporation? Is there any key to how it should act?*

A. Yes. This harks back to my statement that the corporation can't get its charter and then put it on the shelf. The corporation must get a new employer identification number, withhold taxes from the doctors' salaries just as it would for any other employe, and in general make a clean break with the past when the practice functioned as a sole proprietorship or partnership.

Q. *Take a doctor who's used to operating casually. Say he simply grabs $25 or so in cash from the petty cash drawer when he goes to lunch. Will he still be able to do that when he's formed a corporation?*

A. No. Not unless he clearly takes it out as a loan. He'll have to remember that it's not his money, it's the corporation's. The fact that he owns the corporation doesn't make any difference. If he takes the money out that way and doesn't promptly pay it back, then it may count as a dividend. Unlike salary, a dividend is not deductible by a corporation, though it is taxed to the individual.

Q. *Suppose the money was really an advance for a legitimate professional travel or entertainment expense?*

A. As long as the doctor properly accounted to the corporation with a travel or expense voucher that met the legal standards for such accounting, then the money would count as an advance. But I want to emphasize that the doctor must account to the corporation, just the same as any corporate employe must, to be reimbursed for his expenses.

Q. *Some tax practitioners argue that for a smooth transition to a professional corporation, it's necessary to transfer accounts receivable to the corporation. Others claim that if the receivables are transferred, the corporation will have to pay the tax on them as if they'd all been collected on the date of transfer. Will they be treated that way?*

A. Generally, no. If requested, the I.R.S. will ordinarily issue an advance ruling agreeing that the accounts receivable will be considered income only as the corporation collects them, provided two conditions are met: First, the receivables must be transferred to the corporation, and the doctors who "controlled" the prior practice, as defined by the Revenue Code, must also control the corporation. Second, accounts payable must be tranferred to the corporation along with the accounts receivable. If those payables exceed the tax basis of all the assets transferred, including the receivables, there could be special tax problems. But that's not likely in a medical practice.

Q. *Could the doctors pay up their professional debts just before incorporating to get an immediate tax deduction for the payments?*

A. Yes, I think we'd have a hard time finding fault with a man who paid his debts when he could. That assumes those debts would otherwise be deductible when paid, of course. He could not pay debts not yet incurred. For instance, he couldn't pay the rent in advance and then claim a deduction. However, as previously noted, if taxpayers want a ruling that the corporation and not the individuals will be taxable on receivables, they ordinarily will be required to transfer all remaining debts, as well as receivables.

Q. *Another problem that has worried tax practitioners is the matter of the "reasonableness" of a doctor's salary. Some fear that if a doctor earns too much, the I.R.S. may say that some of his income is really a dividend. That would result in double taxation because the payment wouldn't be allowed as a corporate deduction, so it would be taxed once to the corporation and then taxed again as part of the doctor's income. Is there any basis for that fear?*

A. If a doctor has a history of high earnings from his services before forming the corporation, there's no reason why he can't earn the same compensation for his services as an employe of the corporation. But there's another problem: the earnings attributable to the capital investment in his practice. In an individual or partnership practice, he generally had no reason to allocate earnings between capital and services because, from a tax standpoint, it made no difference.

Q. *How would incorporation change things?*

A. Let's say that an individual had been earning $50,000 a year and that he had equipment and goodwill with a market value of $100,000. When he incorporated, he couldn't say that he had been earning $50,000 entirely from his services. He would be earning something on the capital, too.

Q. *How much would the I.R.S. be likely to allocate earnings on capital?*

A. In today's market, where interest goes up to 10 per cent on a loan, the return on an equity investment—that's how the capital is considered—ought to be perhaps 15 per cent or more. If the doctor had the only physiotherapy center around, he might be considered a monopoly and a more normal return in that situation might be 25 or 30 per cent, or even more. So the earnings on capital in the hypothetical case I posed might be at least $15,000 and could exceed $30,000.

Q. *How would allocation of part of the earnings to invested capital affect the doctor's tax situation?*

A. Drastically. The earnings on equity would count as the corporation's and be taxed at that level and then they'd be taxed again as a dividend when the doctor got them. If they counted as compensation, they'd only be taxed once, and part could be diverted into a retirement plan where they'd be exempt from current taxes.

Q. *If a corporation was in a lower tax bracket than a doctor-shareholder, could the doctor accumulate the money in the corporation and avoid the second tax by not paying it out?*

A. Yes, but there's a limit. The law permits a corporation generally to hold profits only up to $150,000. Once a corporation accumulates more profit than that, it's subject to a special high penalty tax unless it can show it's going to need the money for the business.

Q. *Putting all the legal problems aside, what is your personal view of the formation of professional corporations?*

A. As a professional man, I'm concerned about the tendency of doctors, dentists, lawyers, architects, and others to form corporations. I don't think it's necessarily in the public interest. The difficulty arose because sole owners and partners haven't been treated like other taxpayers for retirement plan purposes, but the Treasury has a great deal of interest in making changes in the law relating to deferred compensation so that all similarly situated taxpayers will be treated alike, no matter what the form of their business.

Now that the changes have taken place, incorporated doctors who decide to go back to practicing as individuals or in partnerships could find themselves facing serious tax problems when they start breaking up the corporations they've formed.

18 How They Thwarted a Sneak Attack on Solo Corporations

Long after the battle for professional corporations had been won the Internal Revenue Service still had no clearly-stated policy on solo corporations. Taking his cue from that, an agent in Maine decided that such a corporation "did not possess a sufficient number of the corporate characteristics to qualify for filing as a corporation," and disallowed some $35,000 that had been contributed to the pension plan of the Higgins Professional Association, formed in 1970 by George Higgins, a Presque Isle, Maine, OBG man.

With that action, the I.R.S. auditor had raised a real possibility that many, if not all of the tens of thousands of one-man corporations could have been put out of action—something many corporate experts had feared all along.

After getting the agent's notice, George Higgins, and his tax adviser, Israel S. Laeger, a Bangor, Maine, C.P.A., checked other professional corporations in the area and found that many others had been attacked. Fearing an all-out drive against solos, they looked for expert help.

A call to Medical Economics quickly led them to attorneys Harry V. Lamon Jr. of Atlanta, and Converse Murdoch of Wilmington, Del. They assembled much of the same legal talent that had won the battles for professional corporations in the 60s. With the help of this group, Laeger first asked for "technical advice." That's a procedure that gets an agent's action reviewed in Washington. It's used when there's a belief that an agent is not following correct I.R.S. policy. That's exactly what the national office found when it ruled against the agent. With that, the ghost that had lurked in the background of one-man corporations appears to have been laid to rest once and for all.

The Higgins case brief went thoroughly into the background of the old professional corporation battles. The central theme, however, was simple: state laws, cases, and the I.R.S. made no distinction between a one-man corporation and a multi-man corporation.

One interesting sidelight of the Higgins case is the re-emphasis on the need for a professional corporation to adhere to the niceties of form—something Higgins couldn't be faulted on. The agent himself stated: "No issue is being raised as to failure to adhere to corporate formalities or failure to operate as a corporation."

The sad fact is that many professional corporations remain vulnerable on that point. The recent I.R.S. action may provide a bulwark that even the toughest agent couldn't batter down when it comes to their right to have a one-man corporation, but sloppy corporate minutes and other seemingly petty matters could provide a different opening for a successful attack on any professional corporation.

index